Springer Series on Behavior Therapy and Behavioral Medicine

Series Editors: Cyril M. Franks, Ph.D.
Frederick J. Evans, Ph.D.

Advisory Board: John Paul Brady, M.D., Robert P. Liberman, M.D.,
Neal E. Miller, Ph.D., and Stanley Rachman, Ph.D.

Editor

Richard K. Goodstein, M.D., is Director of Education, Carrier Foundation, Belle Mead, New Jersey, and is Associate Clinical Professor of Psychiatry, Rutgers Medical School. He has written and lectured widely on the topics of medical student education, resident training in psychiatry, agoraphobia, and gerontology.

Contributors

Kelly D. Brownell, Ph.D., is Associate Professor of Psychiatry, University of Pennsylvania School of Medicine, Philadelphia.

Hilde Bruch, M.D., is Professor Emeritus of Psychiatry, Baylor College of Medicine, Houston, Texas.

C. N. Chen, M.Sc., M.B., is Senior Lecturer in Psychiatry, St. George's Hospital Medical School, University of London.

Arthur H. Crisp, D.Sc., M.D., is Professor of Psychiatry, St. George's Hospital Medical School, University of London.

Frederick J. Evans, Ph.D., is Director of Research at Carrier Foundation, Belle Mead, New Jersey, and Adjunct Professor of Psychiatry, Rutgers Medical School, Piscataway, New Jersey.

Cyril M. Franks, Ph.D., is Professor of Psychology, Graduate School of Applied and Professional Psychology, Rutgers University, and Consultant in Clinical Psychology to Carrier Foundation, Belle Mead, New Jersey.

L. K. G. Hsu, M.D., is Lecturer in Psychiatry at St. George's Hospital Medical School, University of London.

Charles Solow, M.D., is Professor of Clinical Psychiatry and Vice Chairman, Department of Psychiatry, Dartmouth College Medical School, Hanover, New Hampshire.

Albert J. Stunkard, M.D., is Professor of Psychiatry, University of Pennsylvania School of Medicine, Philadelphia.

Robert A. Vigersky, M.D., is Staff Endocrinologist, Walter Reed Army Medical Center, Washington, D.C., and Associate Professor of Medicine, Uniformed Services University of the Health Sciences, Bethesda, Maryland.

M. Wheeler, Ph.D., is Principal Biochemist, Department of Chemical Pathology, St. Thomas' Hospital, London.

EATING AND WEIGHT DISORDERS

Advances in Treatment and Research

Richard K. Goodstein, M.D., Editor

SPRINGER PUBLISHING COMPANY
New York

Acknowledgment

The editor wishes to express his appreciation for the dedicated logistical efforts of his secretary, Stephanie Schmitter. The long hours that she devoted to typing and proofreading are of fundamental importance to this book and deserve early and appropriate recognition.

Springer Publishing Company, Inc.
200 Park Avenue South
New York, New York 10003

83 84 85 86 87 / 10 9 8 7 6 5 4 3 2 1

Library of Congress Cataloging in Publication Data

Main entry under title:

Eating and weight disorders.

    (Springer series on behavior therapy and behavioral medicine; 8)
    Includes bibliographical references and index.
    1. Obesity.   2. Obesity—Psychological aspects.   3. Food habits. I. Goodstein, Richard K. II. Series. [DNLM: 1. Obesity—Therapy. 2. Anorexia nervosa—Therapy. 3. Behavior therapy. W1 SP 685NB v.8 / WD 210 E14]
RC628.E28   616.3'98   82–5745
ISBN 0–8261–3830–6   AACR2
ISSN 0278–6729

Printed in the United States of America

Contents

Foreword

This volume presents a most up-to-date account of current knowledge of weight control usefully integrated in one source. Based on extensive research in a number of different areas, a group of experts in the field of weight disorders have pooled their knowledge in order to present the current state-of-the-art understanding of the complex multi-dimensional factors involved in obesity, sudden weight change, anorexia, and related medical problems.

The reader can best appreciate the profound implications for the understanding and management of eating disorders presented here by carefully studying the overview of the biological and psychological determinants of weight control outlined in the first chapter, by Stunkard, summarizing much of the recent evidence concerning food regulation and set points. He provides a solid, empirical underpinning for the many factors that are involved in the psychological, behavioral, physiological, and surgical management of those biological disturbances associated with weight difficulties.

Two major themes are developed throughout this volume. The first is that, for those suffering from overweight and obesity and those with related weight problems such as anorexia, no simple solution is yet available. The clinician looking for some new answer or broadly applicable treatment method is going to be disappointed. Nevertheless, as all contributors make clear, new advances in the management of weight disorders derived from a solid, empirical foundation and based on a careful understanding of all of the metabolic, biological, psychological, and behavioral determinants of these disorders are being developed and evaluated. These advances promise cautious optimism for the future, and it is a privilege to be at the frontier of these new scientific developments.

The second theme is the healthy eclecticism that the contributors maintain in their scientific perspectives and treatment recommendations. There is a multidisciplinary juxtaposition ranging from surgical management of obesity to detailed description and evaluations of strictly behavioral methods and therapeutic communities. The current status of metabolic changes associated with weight loss is presented comfortably along with psychoanalytic and behavioral orientations to understanding both obesity and anorexia. The reader may be surprised to discover that one of the pioneers of behavioral approaches to obesity, and an instigator of the modestly successful self-help weight control programs, summarizes successful outcome research ranging from pharmacological intervention to psychoanalytic treatment.

Those who were able to participate in the Carrier Foundation Twentieth Annual Symposium on Eating and Weight Disorders, which brought together most of these contributors for an intensive consideration of these problems, will be delighted that the proceedings have been expanded into this book. Those who were not fortunate enough to have participated personally in this event will nevertheless appreciate the clinical sensitivity and compassion that these investigators bring to this difficult and frustrating area.

Frederick J. Evans, Ph.D.
Cyril M. Franks, Ph.D.

Preface

All of us identify with food, eating, and weight in one manner or another. Perhaps for this reason an especially enthusiastic response was apparent when the contributors to this book participated as faculty speakers in the 1980 Carrier Foundation Twentieth Annual Symposium on Eating and Weight Disorders.

The key ingredient to this exciting education session was the energetic involvement of these internationally renowned authorities. While some of the faculty presented a comprehensive review of a topic, others offered specific new scientific data. All provided practical advice to clinicians, therapists, and patients.

It is my special delight to share with you expanded portions of the contributors' scholarly work. The book is not intended as a text. Rather, it is a sampling of current topics and developments in the field of eating and weight disorders that have relevance to a wide cross section of the health care professions. A companion book to be published by Springer Publishing Company will highlight the topic of bulimia. Edited by William J. Fremouw, Ph.D., and entitled *Binge Eating: Theory, Research, and Treatment,* it will feature two of our book's contributors and add to the range of information in this volume.

I now wish you good reading, eating, and weight control.

R.K.G.

1
Biological and Psychological Factors in Obesity

Albert J. Stunkard

The treatment of obesity today is based upon an increasingly thorough understanding of the biological and psychological factors that determine this disorder. This was not always the case. For many years the treatment of obesity was purely empirical, and clinicians were forced to rely on a trial-and-error approach, in effect reinventing the wheel with each new patient. For until very recently the knowledge base was lacking. Even 20 years ago a consideration of biological and psychological factors in human obesity might well have been confined to a description of the metabolic derangements of obese people, derangements that have since been shown to be simple consequences of the obese state. A discussion of psychological factors might have been limited to "deep oral problems," problems that have eluded definition as perversely as they have eluded therapy. And any attempt to relate the biological and the psychological—an unlikely event—would have left us as baffled as were readers of Felix Deutsch's book *On the Mysterious Leap from the Mind to the Body* (1959). In other words, we did not know much.

Today all of this has changed. In the past 20 years we have learned a good bit about the biology and psychology of obesity, and what we have learned from one has illuminated the other. The boundaries that used to be so firmly drawn between obesity of psychological origin and obesity of biological origin are fading, and with their fading a paradox has emerged. We know a surprising amount about psychological factors among persons whose obesity is of clearly biological origin.

In this chapter we will describe a theory that relates the biological origins of obesity to some psychological factors, including three common and serious problems in the treatment of obesity, and an intriguing new psychological idea. The theory deals with the regulation of body weight or, more properly, body fat. The first problem is the tendency of obese patients to drop out of treatment for obesity. The second problem is the emotional disturbance that so often afflicts obese people when they diet. The third problem is the strong tendency of obese people to regain the weight lost during treatment. The new psychological idea deals with the distinctive behavioral characteristics of so-called restrained eaters, persons who voluntarily restrict their food intake in order to maintain their body weight at a lower level than it would otherwise be.

Lest it appear that this chapter is unduly preoccupied with problems in the treatment of obesity, it will close with good news from the treatment front. Brief accounts will be given of new developments in the treatment of obesity by psychoanalysis, pharmacotherapy, surgery, and behavior therapy.

The Regulation of Body Weight

Discussions of the biology of body weight have traditionally begun with what seemed a truism: Obesity is the result of a disorder in the regulation of body weight. In experimental animals, at least, nothing seemed more evident than that obesity resulted from a disordered physiological regulation. Animals of normal weight clearly regulate their weight with great precision. Animals with lesions of the ventromedial hypothalamus lose this capacity and, as a consequence, become obese. Or so it seemed.

The evidence for the regulation in animals of normal weight is clear and unequivocal (Keesey, 1980). First, their body weight remains stable (or increases at a constant rate) under normal circumstances. Second, after their body weight has been altered by a variety of experimental manipulations, it returns promptly and predictably to its previous level. Thus, the body weight of animals can be elevated by tube-feeding, by the injection of long-acting insulin, by the establishment of a shock-avoidance-by-eating paradigm or by the use of a high-fat diet. When these conditions are removed, the animals apparently automatically restrict food intake sufficiently to reduce their body weight to pre-experimental levels. Similarly, lowering body weight by starvation is followed by a prompt return to baseline levels when animals are permitted free access to food (Hamilton, 1969).

Establishing the existence of the regulation of body weight is, thus, quite straightforward. It consists of nothing more than determining that animals can return body weight to pre-experimental levels after the experimental conditions that change it are removed. Once regulation is viewed in this light it becomes simple enough to ask whether obese animals also regulate body weight. Hoebel and Teitelbaum (1966) were the first to ask, and they answered it with an emphatic "yes." Figure 1.1 depicts their experiment with a rat made hyperphagic and obese by lesions in the ventromedial hypothalamus. Once the body weight of the animal leveled off, the introduction of forced feeding resulted in a prompt increase in body weight. Termination of forced feeding brought about a compensatory fall in food intake sufficient to restore body weight to pre-experimental levels. Similarly, starvation for a period of 20 days resulted in marked loss of weight. Free access to food was followed by an increase in food intake and restoration of body weight to its prestarvation level.

The hypothalamic obese rat thus meets the criteria for the regulation of body weight. But if its regulation is not impaired, why is the rat obese? Control theory suggests an answer. The "set point" about which

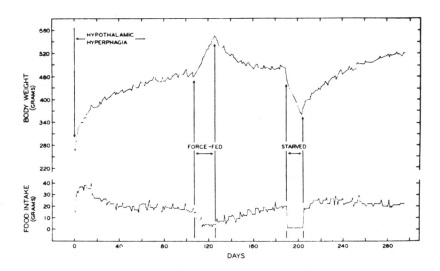

Figure 1.1. Effects of force-feeding and starvation on food intake and body weight of a rat with ventromedial hypothalamic lesions.

From Hoebel, R. G., & Teitelbaum, P. Weight regulation in normal and hypothalamic rats. *Journal of Comparative and Physiological Psychology*, 1966, *61*, 189–193. Copyright © 1966 by the American Psychological Association. Reprinted by permission.

body weight is regulated is elevated. Weight can thus be higher, but still regulated.

There is good experimental evidence for the regulation of body weight in hypothalamic obese rats and, in fact, in other forms of experimental obesity. Regulation implies the existence of a set point or, as Wirtshafter and Davis (1977) call it, a "settling point." But is there evidence for an elevated set point? Another experiment by Hoebel and Teitelbaum (1966) suggests that there is.

Figure 1.2 shows the production of obesity by means of long-acting insulin injections. When the rat's weight had reached the obese level of 460 grams, the ventromedial nucleus was destroyed bilaterally. Two outcomes were possible: (1) If hypothalamic obesity simply resulted from neural damage releasing the inhibitory influences of satiety areas in the hypothalamus, hyperphagia and an increase in body weight should ensue. (2) If, on the other hand, the body weight of hypothalamic obese animals is regulated by a set point, and if body weight were increased to that level prior to hypothalamic lesions, these

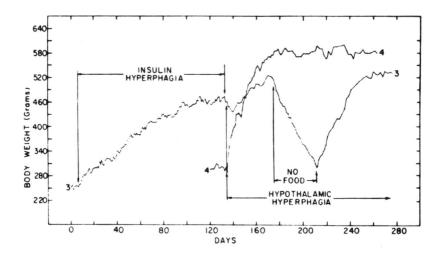

Figure 1.2. Failure of rat to increase body weight following ventromedial hypothalamic lesions when obesity had already been produced by chronic insulin injection. The usual course of increase in body weight following such lesions is seen in the second rat.

From Hoebel, R. G., & Teitelbaum, P. Weight regulation in normal and hypothalamic rats. *Journal of Comparative and Physiological Psychology,* 1966, *61,* 189–193. Copyright © 1966 by the American Psychological Association. Reprinted by permission.

lesions should produce no additional overeating and no further increase in body weight.

The data in Figure 1.2 favor the second alternative. Hypothalamic lesions were followed by only trivial increases in body weight. The existence of a set point at about 460 grams was further substantiated by the return of body weight to this level after it had been reduced by temporary starvation. The usual course of hypothalamic obesity is shown in the weight curve of a second rat, whose normal body weight increased rapidly following hypothalamic lesions.

Since these studies were conducted, evidence has been obtained for a symmetry in the ability to regulate body weight by a study of rats made hypophagic and underweight by lesions in the lateral hypothalamus. Studies by Keesey (1980) have shown that the food intake of rats following lateral hypothalamic lesions is apparently controlled in such a way as to produce a new lower weight level. If lesioned at a normal body weight, these animals were aphagic and achieved their new maintenance level by the loss of body weight. If lesioned when their body weights were *below* the new level, however, the rats were actually hyperphagic for the short period of time necessary to increase their weight to its new level. The primary effect of lateral hypothalamic lesions seems to be to set a new and reduced level of body weight. Changes in food intake seem to be secondary in order to achieve this new level.

What is the relevance of experiments with brain-damaged rats to the problems of human obesity? These are, after all, special experimental preparations. Yet the very fact that they are special argues for their relevance. If damage to not just one, but to two, weight regulatory areas in the hypothalamus does not destroy the ability to regulate body weight, the phenomenon must be robust. And if the phenomenon is found, as it apparently is, in every animal in which it has yet been investigated, our own species can hardly be exempt. Clearly, far more numerous and more complex phenomena determine body weight in humans. But it seems likely that the regulation of body weight underlies these phenomena.

Regulation of Body Weight in Humans

The regulation of body weight has been studied only twice in humans, but both studies strongly suggest that regulation occurs. Each study involved persons of normal weight and each used the standard method for establishing the presence of regulation—perturbing body weight and then removing the perturbation. Keys, Brozek, Henschel, Mickelson, and Taylor (1950) studied the biology of human starvation by subjecting young male volunteers to a 1600-calorie diet that reduced their body weights to 75 percent of their pre-experimental level. When these volunteers were subsequently refed, they overate sufficiently to restore their body weights to their pre-experimental levels. They apparently paid no particular attention to their caloric intake or their body weight in the process.

Sims and Horton (1968) carried out the second study of the regulation of body weight in humans. It showed that normal-weight men could restore body weight after excessive caloric intake. Twenty-two male volunteers were paid to eat a diet containing as many as 8000 calories a day for a period of 40 days. During this time their body weight increased by 15 to 25 percent. Thereafter, when these men were permitted to eat *ad libitum*, they underate for a period of time sufficient to restore their body weights to pre-experimental levels. As after experimental undernutrition, these men paid no attention to either food intake or body weight in order to achieve this result. Thus, two well-designed experiments make it seem likely that persons of normal weight maintain their weight at this level by an active process of regulation.

Nonobese people evidently regulate body weight. Do obese people?

Conventional wisdom has held that obese people do not regulate body weight and that, in fact, the failure of their ability to regulate is the cause of their obesity. There is a sound clinical basis for this belief. Lifetime weight histories of obese persons usually show a very erratic course; it is hard, if not impossible, to find any baseline about which their wide fluctuations in body weight might be regulated. Yet it would be remarkable indeed if obese persons were the only animals who did not possess the capacity to regulate their body weight. Do they really lack this capacity, or do they simply fail to exercise it?

Nisbett (1972) has proposed a theory that may answer this question. According to this theory, obese people may well possess the capacity to regulate body weight. However, they have been biologically programmed to be fat and the set point about which their weight would be regulated by purely physiological forces is higher than that which is tolerated by social pressures. So they diet for cosmetic reasons, thereby reducing their weight below the level at which it would be maintained without this effort. The result is a paradox: persons whose body weights are, despite their obesity, below their physiological set points. In other words, these people are at the same time statistically overweight and biologically underweight! According to this view, much of their distinctive behavior is not a result of their being obese, but of their not being obese enough. Preoccupation with food, increased taste responsiveness, emotionality, physical inactivity, even the elevated levels of free fatty acids in the blood, are all characteristics shared by fat people and starving people. There are striking similarities between the behavior of fat people and that of semistarved volunteers in the study by Keys and co-workers (1950) on the biology of human starvation.

Nisbett proposed that some people are biologically programmed to be fat. Is this a reasonable proposal? How might such programming occur? What might set a set point?

A prominent candidate for the biological basis of obesity is clearly adipose tissue, and recent research on adipose tissue has provided strong support for its role as a determinant of body weight (Sjöström, 1980). The adipose tissue of some obese persons, particularly those whose obesity began early in life—the so-called juvenile-onset obese—may contain more fat cells than does the adipose tissue of either nonobese persons or of persons whose obesity began during adult life. Indeed, the adipose tissue of morbidly obese persons may contain five times as many fat cells as that of persons in the other two categories. As a result, under usual conditions, they not only contain far more fat than do their lean fellows, but when they reduce, the fat content of their individual fat cells must be reduced to one-fifth the size of a "normal" fat cell for them to reach statistically normal levels of body weight. We still do not know the physiological effects of such radical depletion of the fat content of individual fat cells. It does appear, though, that adipose tissue could well constitute the agency for setting a body weight set point. Four very different clinical phenomena support this proposition. Indeed, this proposition that adipose tissue is a major determinant of weight regulation provides the most parsimonious explanation of these four phenomena: (1) dropping out of treatment for obesity, (2) emotional disturbances during dieting, (3) regaining weight lost in treatment, and (4) the new concept of "restrained eating." Research inspired by these newer notions of adipose tissue has shed new light on each of these phenomena in the very recent past. Let us consider this exciting new research.

Three Clinical Problems

Dropping Out of Treatment for Obesity

The most direct evidence relating fat-cell size to a clinical phenomenon has been a Swedish study on dropping out of treatment. Fat-cell size of 26 patients was measured during the course of a traditional weight-reduction regimen that produced an average weight loss of 33 pounds (Björntorp, Carlgren, Isaksson, Krotkiewski, Larsson, & Sjöström, 1975). Figure 1.3 shows the body weight of each patient at the beginning and end of treatment. These values varied widely and reached normal levels at the end of treatment in only ten patients. Most of the rest dropped out of treatment.

Figure 1.4, which relates total body fat to the fat content of individual fat cells, tells a very different story. On the abscissa we see once again a wide variability in body fat content at the time that the patients started and stopped treatment. When we look at fat-cell size as plotted on the ordinate, however, the values at the end of treatment are remarkably similar. Those of 23 of the 26 patients are normal! Figure 1.4 suggests that most patients stopped treatment at widely varying levels of body fat, but at precisely that point when further weight loss could be achieved only by reducing their fat cells to subnormal size. It was as if fat-cell size, perhaps particularly events at the cell membrane, had set a biological limit to weight reduction. This kind of limit should occur in any person with an excessive number of fat cells, for such persons can reduce to statistically normal body weight only by greatly depleting the fat content of their individual fat cells. Such depletion could go far toward explaining the difficulty that many obese persons experience in reducing to a statistically "normal" body weight and their strong tendency to regain the weight that they have lost.

Emotional Disturbances during Dieting

The study of Björntorp and associates (1975) suggests that reducing individual fat-cell size contributes to the problem of dropping out of treatment for obesity. One reason obese people drop out of treatment is that they develop emotional disturbances. These emotional disturbances—the so-called dieting depression—(Stunkard, 1957) are among the most common, baffling, and troublesome clinical features of obesity. Bruch first called attention to the problem in 1952 with her description of two patients who developed such disturbances in the course of dieting. The first systematic assessment was conducted by Stunkard and McLaren-Hume (1959) with 100 consecutive obese patients referred to the nutrition clinic from all parts of a general hospital. The assessment was thus carried out on a relatively unbiased sample. In order to avoid the bias resulting from the high dropout rate of persons suffering from emotional disturbance, patients in this study were not asked about symptoms during their *current* diet, but rather about symptoms during *previous* diets. Seventy-two patients reported pre-

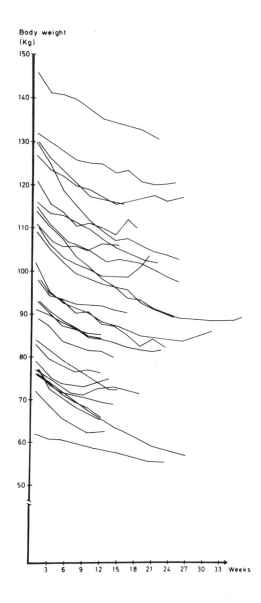

Figure 1.3. Decrease in body weight with time among 28 obese women on reducing diets.

FAT CELL WEIGHT (μg)

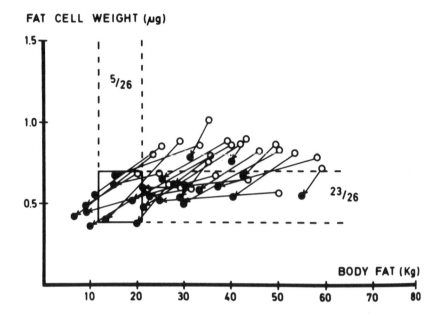

Figure 1.4. Body fat and average fat-cell size in obese women (open symbols) and changes on an energy-reduced diet (arrows and filled symbols). Rectangle denotes mean ± standard deviation of values of controls. Note the consistent fat-cell weight at which patients failed to decrease body weight.

From Björntorp, P., Carlgren, G., Isaksson, B., Krotkiewski, M., Larsson, B., & Sjöstrom, L. Effect of an energy-reduced dietary regimen in relation to adipose tissue cellularity in obese women. *American Journal of Clinical Nutrition,* 1975, *28,* 445–452. Copyright © 1975 by the American Society of Clinical Nutrition. Reprinted with permission.

vious diets and Table 1.1 shows that over half had at least one symptom that they attributed to dieting.

Silverstone and Lascelles (1966) reported the incidence of emotional disturbance during one of the few traditional weight-reduction programs with a dropout rate that was low enough (17 percent) not to unduly bias the outcome. Seventy-two patients started treatment, 60 completed it. Table 1.1 shows that exactly half of these patients reported either onset or intensification of symptoms of depression during treatment. Furthermore, 25 patients reported increases in anxiety and 11 of them became "markedly anxious."

Stunkard and Rush (1974) reviewed the extensive literature on this topic and confirmed the high incidence of emotional disturbance

Table 1.1 Symptoms during Outpatient Dieting

Retrospectively (All Efforts)*		Prospectively (One Diet)†	
Nervousness	21%	Depression	50%
Weakness	21%	Anxiety	40%
Irritability	8%		
Fatigue	5%		
Nausea	4%		
Total Reporting 54%			

*From data collected by Stunkard & McLaren-Hume, 1959.
†From data collected by Silverstone & Lascelles, 1966.

in both inpatients and outpatients treated for obesity. Three variables affect the incidence of these disturbances: (1) Persons with childhood onset of obesity are more vulnerable than those with adult onset of obesity; (2) severe caloric restriction apparently produces symptoms more readily than does a total fast; (3) outpatient treatment appears to be more stressful than inpatient treatment.

Morbidly obese people who diet suffer even more severely from emotional disturbances than do less obese persons. Halmi, Stunkard, and Mason (1980) described the emotional responses to dieting reported by 70 women and 10 men who averaged 137 percent overweight and who later underwent gastric bypass surgery for their obesity. Most of these patients had experienced emotional disturbances during dieting. The commonest complaints were preoccupation with food, irritability, anxiety, and depression. Table 1.2 shows that only a minority had escaped untoward consequences of dieting and that for many these consequences had been "severe."

Table 1.2 Untoward Responses to Previous Weight Loss by Dieting

	Severe	Moderate	Mild	None	Other
Depression	15	26	20	34	5
Anxiety	23	30	20	24	3
Irritability	35	29	16	15	5
Preoccupation with food	53	20	8	15	4

From Halmi, K. A., Stunkard, A. J., & Mason, E. E. Emotional responses to weight reduction by three methods: gastric bypass, jejunoileal bypass, and diet. *American Journal of Clinical Nutrition*, 1980, *33*, 446–451. Copyright © 1980 by the American Society of Clinical Nutrition. Reprinted with permission.

Although the occurrence of emotional disturbances during dieting has been recognized for over 20 years and is among the most firmly established phenomena in the treatment of obesity, we have until recently had no clues as to the origins of these disturbances. Our growing understanding of the anatomy and physiology of adipose tissue now provides such clues. Depletion of the fat content of individual fat cells clearly has important consequences at the cell membrane, consequences that could readily be translated into humoral signals to the central nervous system. The individual fat cells of morbidly obese persons become more extensively depleted as they approach statistically "normal" levels of body weight. Such depletion could well increase the strength of the humoral signals and the consequent intensity of the emotional disturbances of these people. At long last a path to a better understanding of these disturbances may be at hand.

Regaining Weight Lost in Treatment

Weight loss during treatment for obesity is not only associated with emotional disturbances and dropping out of treatment; it is also regularly followed by regaining of the weight lost during treatment. In fact, most obese people regain most of the weight that they lose during treatment. This sequence is particularly well-documented for the weight losses that follow therapeutic fasting. The largest follow-up study of therapeutic fasting is that of Drenick and Johnson (1978), who reported on 121 of 207 patients who had lost large amounts of weight. Data on the others were missing because of "failure to answer the questionnaire, inability to locate patients and death"; presumably the outcome of these missing patients was even poorer than that of those who were studied. Patients were mostly women who were 89 percent overweight, fasted 47 days, and lost 62 pounds. Virtually all regained the weight that they had lost. Figure 1.5 shows that the weight of 50 percent had returned to its initial value in less than three years. Fewer than 10 percent remained below the original level nine years after the fast. There was no difference in rates of regaining to original weight between adult-onset and childhood-onset obese groups. Regaining to more than the original admission weight, however, was more common (42 percent) among childhood-onset than among adult-onset obese persons (26 percent).

Noting that the variability in individual responses to weight reduction is obscured by the use of grouped data, Stunkard and Penick (1979) developed a method for displaying the data of individual pa-

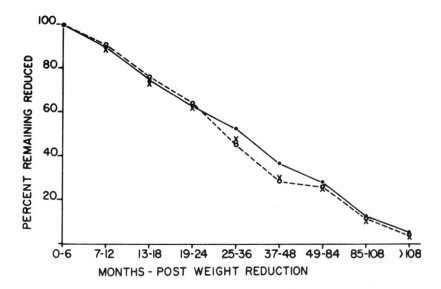

Figure 1.5. Percentage of patients remaining reduced at various time intervals following weight loss. Solid line represents 60 subjects with obesity onset before age 21; the interrupted line represents 42 subjects with obesity onset after age 21. The ×-symbols represent the experience of the entire group.

From Drenick, E. J., & Johnson, D. Weight reduction by fasting and semistarvation in morbid obesity: Long-term follow-up. *International Journal of Obesity*, 1978, *2*, 123–132. Copyright © 1978 by John Libby & Co. Ltd. Reprinted by permission of the author and the publisher.

tients. Weight loss at the end of treatment is plotted on the horizontal axis of Figure 1.6 and weight loss at follow-up (initial weight − follow-up weight) on the vertical axis. Data points of patients who simply maintained the weight they had lost during treatment thus fall along the main diagonal. Continuing weight loss after the end of treatment is represented by data points above the main diagonal, continuing weight gain by points below it.

We applied this method to Swanson and Dinello's study (1970) of the results of therapeutic fasting. Figure 1.6 shows the remarkable degree to which the weights of individual patients fell below the main diagonal, representing the regaining of weight following treatment. Note further the striking linearity of these data points along the horizontal axis, attesting to the precision of return to baseline following weight losses of very different magnitudes. This phenomenon clearly suggests an active process of regulation.

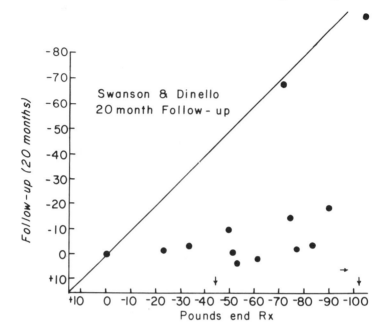

Figure 1.6. Figure plotted from data published in Swanson & Dinello (1970). See text for explanation of method. Note the consistency with which weight returns to baseline after treatment.

A Clinical Theory

"Restrained Eating"

Nisbett's theory that the body weight of some obese people is below a set point helps to explain three serious problems in the management of obesity: dropping out of treatment, emotional disturbances during dieting, and the tendency to regain weight lost during treatment. This explanation of these diverse phenomena is valuable in itself, and the power of the explanation supports this theory. But it is, in a sense, *post hoc* support. The strength of a scientific theory, however, is determined less by its explanatory power than by its predictive power. By this criterion, Nisbett's theory is seriously flawed: it cannot be tested directly. Such a test would require that we know the body weight set point of individual people, let them gain to this level and then see if they regulate. The test fails on two grounds, ethical and scientific. Ethically, we are not justified in such a test; scientifically, we do not know the body weight set points of individual people and we cannot find them out.

Nisbett's theory cannot be tested directly, but it can be tested indirectly, and Herman has done precisely this (Herman & Mack, 1975; Herman & Polivy, 1975, 1980). Reasoning that anyone who is consciously keeping his weight below set point should be able to tell you so, he asked people. Were they trying to restrain the amount they ate? For this purpose he used an 11-item "restrained eating" questionnaire. People identified as "restrained eaters" by this questionnaire appear to have distinctive behavioral responses, quite different from those of "unrestrained eaters"—people who can eat almost anything they want and still maintain their body weight. For example, when given a pre-load of food in a taste testing experiment, restrained eaters will eat *more* food in performing the test while unrestrained eaters, who regulate body weight normally, eat less. Under appropriate laboratory circumstances, alcohol increased the food intake of restrained eaters but not that of unrestrained eaters. Restrained eaters tend to gain weight when they are depressed, in contrast to the loss of weight during depression, which is the more common outcome. Finally, a recently published report indicates that the concept of restrained eating actually includes three quite separate factors—restraint itself, disinhibition of restraint, and hunger (Stunkard, 1981). The usefulness of this distinction has been increased by a study of the relationship of these three factors to adipose tissue cellularity. Whereas fat cell number correlates highly with disinhibition of restraint, fat cell size correlates with restraint itself (Stunkard, 1981). It appears that for restrained eaters the pressures to conform to the slim ideal of beauty are stronger than the biological pressures generated by adipose tissue.

The experimental methods used by Herman derive from those of his mentor, Stanley Schachter (1971), who carried out some of the first studies of human eating behavior in the laboratory. Schachter's research led to the formulation of his well-known "externality" hypothesis. This hypothesis states that obese people are *more* responsive to "external" food cues in the environment than are people of normal weight, and, conversely, obese people are *less* responsive to "internal," physiological, cues to eating. Herman has proposed that most of the behavior that Schachter had ascribed to obesity is not due to obesity but to restraint in eating. According to this view, the findings with obese people were due to the fact that they are more likely to be restrained eaters than are nonobese people.

Some of the experiments upon which Herman has based his restrained eating theory are essentially replications of experiments that Schachter had used to support his externality theory. Early in this research Schachter, Goldman, and Gordon (1968) reported that if obese people consumed a preload of sandwiches and soft drinks, they subsequently ate *more* test food than they did without the preload. Nonobese people, on the other hand, ate less following the preload. This difference in results was an important part of the early support for externality theory. Herman and Mack (1975) repeated this experiment in modified form, investigating restrained/unrestrained eater differences rather than obese/nonobese differences. They reasoned that the failure to manifest short-term regulation, which Schachter had ascribed to obese people, was actually a function of the dietary restraint of these people. Herman and Mack gave their subjects preloads of either two glasses of milkshake, one glass, or none. Then they measured the amount that the subjects ate in what was explained to them as an ice cream–testing experiment. Figure 1.7 shows that, as expected, restrained eaters ate less ice cream than did unrestrained eaters when asked to taste-test ice cream without a preload. After one milkshake, unrestrained eaters, also as expected, ate less ice cream. Restrained eaters, on the other hand, ate *more* following the preload of one milkshake. Furthermore, this difference between restrained and unrestrained eaters became even greater with a preload of two milkshakes. Unrestrained eaters, manifesting appropriate regulation, ate less following one milkshake; restrained eaters ate even more than after one milkshake, demonstrating what Herman has called "counterregulation."

What is the nature and significance of this counterregulation? Herman has suggested that when normally restrained eaters suspend their self-imposed restraint, they come face to face with a state of chronic caloric deprivation. Having abandoned the hope of staying within the caloric limits that they had set for themselves, they give in to the demands of the hunger that they had been suppressing. Further preloading experiments have confirmed the usefulness of "restrained eating" as a predictor of behavior and have dissected the relative contributions of hunger and of disinhibition to this phenomenon. Although both factors play a part, cognitive elements—disinhibition— are more important than are physiological ones.

Restrained eating is also related to depression. Two aspects of the classical picture of depression are anorexia and weight loss. Yet some people eat more, not less, when they are depressed, and gain weight rather than losing it. What is the explanation for these diametrically opposite responses? Herman and Polivy (1975) relate it to the character of the patient's eating prior to the onset of depression. According to

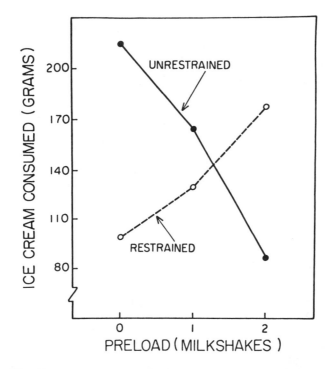

Figure 1.7. Response to preload in restrained and unrestrained eaters.
From Herman, C. P., & Polivy, J. Restrained eating. In A. J. Stunkard (Ed.), *Obesity*. Philadelphia: Saunders, 1980, pp. 208–225. Copyright © 1980 by Saunders Publishing Co. Reprinted by permission of the author and the publisher.

this view, it is the unrestrained eater (who normally regulates body weight without difficulty) who shows the classical pattern of anorexia and weight loss during depression. By contrast, restrained eaters eat more and gain weight when they are depressed. Herman proposes that depression, like preloading in the experiment, disinhibits restraint. The restrained eater who becomes depressed thereby loses his cognitive controls over eating and biological pressures to eat force body weight up to the level for which it had been biologically programmed. A study of 12 mildly depressed people provides empirical support for this plausible hypothesis (Herman & Polivy, 1975). A study, recently completed, of 45 persons suffering from major depression, has confirmed this finding (Weissenburger, Rush, Giles, Kumetz, & Stunkard, in press).

A final piece of evidence supporting the idea of restrained eating, and its relevance to the biology of obesity, has recently been obtained (Stunkard, 1981). A new and expanded restrained eating questionnaire was administered to 55 obese people whose fat-cell size and number had been measured. The predicted relationship was found: the higher the score on both the restrained eating and the hunger scales of the questionnaire, the smaller the size of the person's fat cells.

An understanding of the regulation of body weight helps to delineate some of the biological boundaries of obesity. The treatment of obesity must be carried out within certain biological constraints. Prominent among these restraints is an efficient weight regulatory capacity, which helps to explain such problems as the emotional disturbance that so often accompanies weight loss and the weight gain that so often follows it.

The Bright Side of the Problems

Here surely is a tale of woe. This nice, tidy regulatory theory does not seem to leave a lot of hope for fat people or for the doctors who are trying to help them. But before the reader abandons all hope, let us reconsider. Things are not as bad as they seem. Consider, for instance, the bright side of the very problems that we have just discussed.

First, although many obese patients do drop out of treatment, most do not, and the advent of behavior therapy has decreased still further the number of patients who drop out of treatment.

Second, although emotional disturbances during dieting are common, large numbers of people do not experience them and many even feel better as they lose weight. Behavior therapy has also introduced an element of hope to this problem. Behavioral weight reduction programs have never reported the same amount of emotional disturbance as have traditional dietary programs. And quite recently Craighead, Stunkard, and O'Brien (1981) have reported significant improvement in mental health indices, both at the end of a behavioral weight-reduction program and one year later.

Third, although regaining of weight lost during treatment is a serious problem, it is not universal. Some people have always maintained weight losses and more of them are succeeding with the newer treatments. Behavior therapy produces far better maintenance of weight loss with mild to moderate obesity than does pharmacotherapy (Craighead et al., 1981), and surgical treatments have had even greater success with morbid obesity.

Fourth, even the restrained-eating story offers grounds for hope.

Only some obese people are restrained eaters, who are already exerting their maximum effort to control their food intake. Many obese people are unrestrained eaters, or only partly restrained eaters, and they still have considerable capacity for restraint left. They can do better than they have been in controlling their weight. And many are doing just that, with the help of the new developments in treatment described below.

Here, then, is the good news. But how does it square with the regulatory theory that has just been proposed? How do these patients defy the regulation of body weight that inexorably constrains the treatment of so many obese patients?

The answer is simple. The fine theory, as we noted in the introduction, probably applies to only some obese people, perhaps no more than a minority. Obesity is a disorder involving a physiological regulation—the regulation of energy balance. It may be no more specific than other disorders involving regulations—the regulation of body temperature, for example. Just as there may be all kinds of fevers, there may be all kinds of obesity. It is quite likely that the problems that we have described are peculiar only to certain types of obesity. We have as yet no nosology of the obesities nor even any factual basis for constructing one. It may be years before we know enough to provide an account of all the different possible kinds of obesity. But we may just know more about the kind of obesity that gives rise to the problems that we have discussed than we do about other possible kinds of obesity, for it seems likely that these particular problems occur in people whose adipose tissue contains an excessively large number of fat cells—so-called hyperplastic obesity. The problems we have discussed may be largely problems of this minority of obese persons.

The Good News:
New Treatments for Obesity

Whatever the theoretical basis for problems in the treatment of obesity, there are practical grounds for hope. The good news is that there is considerable progress in the treatment of obesity. I will briefly mention four areas in which progress has been made. They are psychological, pharmacological, behavioral, and surgical.

It may come as something of a surprise to learn that a new area of psychological treatment is an old standby: psychoanalysis.

Psychoanalysis

It has been many years since psychoanalysis has been proposed as a treatment for obesity, and even then there were few such proposals and they were tentative at best. Analysts themselves have been skeptical of the value of psychoanalysis for obesity, and no more than 6 percent of obese persons who enter psychoanalysis do so for treatment of their obesity.

This pessimism may have been premature. Ten years ago the American Academy of Psychoanalysis authorized a study of obese patients in psychoanalysis with members of the Academy (Rand & Stunkard, 1977, 1978). Seventy-two analysts pooled information on 84 of their obese patients over a period of five years. What has emerged from this study has been surprising and promising.

First, consider weight loss. The results of psychoanalysis compare very favorably with those of other conservative (nonsurgical) treatments for obesity. Average weight loss was 21 pounds during treatment that averaged 42 months in duration. Furthermore, this average weight loss was not the result of a few patients who lost a great deal of weight; it was well distributed across all patients in treatment. As Figure 1.8 shows, 47 percent of patients lost more than 20 pounds and 19 percent lost more than 40 pounds.

This amount of weight loss during psychoanalysis came as a distinct surprise. Less surprising, perhaps, but equally gratifying was the improvement among patients who suffered from body-image disparagement. Although most obese persons are at least somewhat concerned about their appearance, for a minority, this concern attains pathological intensity, filling their waking hours with obsessive preoccupation with their weight. Such persons consider their own bodies as grotesque and loathesome and believe that others can view them only with hostility and contempt (Stunkard & Mendelson, 1967). Severe disparagement of the body image is a chronic, intractable disorder, strongly resistant to change and ameliorated only temporarily by weight loss. It is therefore worthy of note that many patients reported striking decreases in the intensity of their body-image disparagment. At the beginning of treatment 40 percent reported severe body-image disparagement; at termination of treatment this figure had fallen to 14 percent.

These favorable results of treatment occurred despite the fact that obese patients were harder to treat than nonobese patients. For example, more obese than nonobese patients terminated treatment prematurely and those who remained in treatment showed less improvement in psychological functioning.

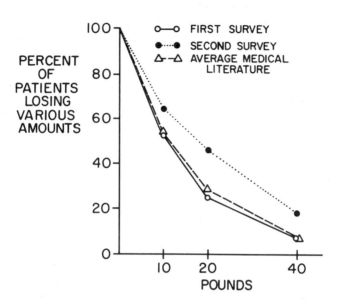

CUMULATIVE WEIGHT LOSSES

Figure 1.8. Cumulative weight losses of obese psychoanalytic patients and obese patients seen in general practice. First survey done after means of 18 months of treatment, second survey at 42 months.

From Rand, C. S. W., & Stunkard, A. J., Obesity and Psychoanalysis. *American Journal of Psychiatry*, 1978, *135*, 547–551. Copyright © 1978 by American Psychiatric Association. Reprinted by permission of the publisher.

Psychoanalysis is an expensive form of treatment and it is not likely that even the favorable results reported here will move large numbers of obese persons to the psychoanalytic couch. Most obese persons will surely seek more economical treatments, at least at the beginning. But for persons who have repeatedly failed with other treatments for obesity, who have the necessary psychological and financial endowment, and particularly for those who have associated neurotic problems, psychoanalysis can now be viewed as a reasonable option.

Pharmacological Treatment

Pharmacological treatment of obesity usually means use of the traditional appetite suppressants; here there is nothing new. There is, however, something new in the treatment of a very special disorder—

bulimia. Bulimia, or binge-eating, afflicts nonobese as well as obese people. Although many people report that they "binge" during Thanksgiving dinners, they are usually not referring to true bulimia. Bulimia is a disorder of far greater intensity. It consists of the impulsive, unpredictable, episodic, and rapid ingestion of large amounts of food during short periods of time. The episode does not usually terminate until the onset of physical discomfort such as abdominal pain, and it may be followed by self-induced vomiting. Patients report feelings of guilt, remorse, and self-contempt after the episode. Bulimia is a chronic, intractable disorder that may go into temporary remission. It occurs in persons of widely varying weights—those with anorexia nervosa, those of normal weight, and those who are obese. The body weight of bulimics is determined not only by the number and severity of the binges but also by the amount of associated vomiting and of other food intake. Bulimia is a source of great distress. Treatment, usually psychotherapy, is generally ineffective.

In 1974 Green and Rau reported an uncontrolled study in which nine of ten "compulsive eaters" experienced marked relief from the use of the anticonvulsant phenytoin in standard therapeutic doses. Although the nature of the "compulsive eating" was not described, it seems probable that it constituted bulimia. Accordingly, Wermuth, Davis, Hollister, and Stunkard (1977) conducted a double-blind, placebo-controlled study of the most severe bulimic women that could be found in a very large population. Ten patients were of normal weight, four were overweight (10 to 20 percent by standard tables), five were obese (more than 20 percent overweight), and one had active anorexia nervosa. Phenytoin was administered in doses of 100 mg of phenytoin three times a day, and a largely successful effort was made to maintain serum levels of phenytoin between 10 and 20 μg/ml.

The frequency of binges was reduced from 3.7 ± 1.9 to 2.3 ± 1.9 for the group as a whole, with great variability in response. Eight of the 19 patients who completed treatment were greatly benefited, six decreasing the frequency of their binges by 75 percent or more and two by 50 to 75 percent. The 11 others were benefited little or not at all. One surprising finding was the persistence of treatment effects for a period of several weeks following discontinuation of medication in most patients who had benefited from it. Two of four patients who continued phenytoin after termination of the study had no further binges during an 18-month follow-up period. Two others reported a return of binges despite continuing treatment and discontinued medication.

Phenytoin is an effective treatment for some severe bulimics, as many as one-third of whom may achieve significant relief from this medication.

Behavior Therapy for Children

The third major new development in treatment for obesity is behavior therapy. Dr. Brownell's chapters describe this modality in some detail and I will not preempt his message. But I will briefly describe some recent research that should improve behavioral weight-reduction programs for children.

As Dr. Brownell notes, behavioral weight control of children has lagged behind that of adults; only recently have there been carefully controlled studies of children. These studies have shown surprising promise. This promise is the more remarkable in that far less is known about the behavior of obese children than about the behavior of obese adults. We have not known, for example, whether they eat too much or exercise too little, or both. A rational behavioral treatment requires this information. A very recent study has provided it; obese children eat too much (Waxman & Stunkard, 1980). Physical inactivity probably does not seriously contribute to their obesity.

Questions about the determinants of obesity in children have been with us for a long time. Bruch (1940) was the first to study these questions systematically. Forty years ago she reported that obese children ate more than nonobese children, a conclusion to which we are finally returning. Unfortunately, four subsequent studies found no difference between obese and nonobese children (Cahn, 1968; Maxfield & Konishi, 1966; Stefanic, Heald, & Mayer, 1959; Wilkinson, Parklin, Pearloom, Strong, & Sykes, 1977). All of these studies were based only upon parental reports, not measurements of behavior and they are, therefore, subject to serious bias.

Similar uncertainty has existed regarding the physical activity of obese children. It is widely believed that obese children are less active than nonobese children and even that inactivity may cause their obesity. Much of this evidence, however, is also based on parental reports. One oft-quoted study that used a more objective measure—motion picture sampling—did find that obese girls were less active than nonobese girls (Bullen, Reed, & Mayer, 1964). But four other studies that utilized objective measures—pedometers or continuous heart-rate monitoring—failed to reveal significant differences between the activity of obese and nonobese children (Bradfield, Paulos, & Grossman,

1971; Maxfield & Konishi, 1966; Stunkard & Pestka, 1962; Wilkinson et al., 1977).

In an effort to avoid the limitations imposed by reliance on parental reports, Waxman and Stunkard (1980) directly measured caloric intake and energy expenditure of children in four families during meals and at play in three different settings. Subjects were four obese boys, and controls were their four brothers, less than two years apart in age. The results were unequivocal: obese boys consumed more calories than their nonobese brothers, and they also *expended* somewhat more calories (Figure 1.9).

The obese boys consumed more calories (766) than did their nonobese controls at supper (504) and far more calories (907) than their controls at lunch (500). The obese boys also ate faster at dinner (65.7 vs. 31.7 kcal/minute) and much faster at school (103.5 vs. 46.2 kcal/minute).

Time-sampled assessment of activity showed that the obese boys were far less active inside the home, slightly less active outside the home, and equally active at school. Oxygen consumption of the boys at four levels of physical activity permitted the calculation of caloric expenditure from the measures of observed activity. These calculations changed the picture dramatically. The obese boys expended more energy per unit of activity than did their controls. Consequently, there was no difference in energy expenditure between obese and nonobese boys inside the home, while the obese boys actually expended more energy outside the home and in school. These findings must be confirmed with larger samples and with girls, but there is now good reason to believe that the basic problem of obese children is that they eat too much. This knowledge makes it easier to construct treatment programs for obese children.

Surgical Treatments for Obesity

The fourth major new development in the treatment of obesity is surgery, directed toward massive, morbid obesity, 100 percent and more above ideal weight. Although the prevalence of morbid obesity is very low—less than one percent—over half a million Americans suffer from it and many of them seek psychiatric treatment at some time in their lives. It is, therefore, useful for psychiatrists to know something about surgical treatment of this disorder. Dr. Solow discusses these treatments in greater detail in chapter 2, and he is just the person to do

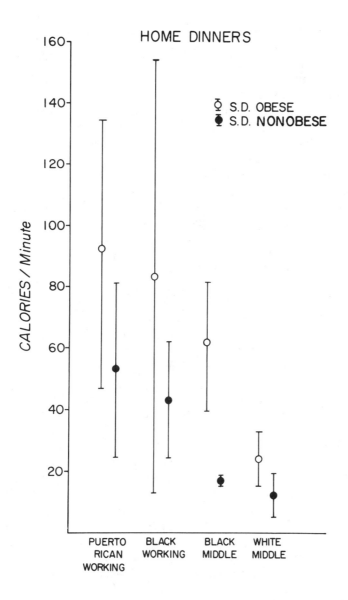

Figure 1.9. Significantly greater caloric intake by obese boys at home dinners as compared with that of their nonobese brothers.

From Waxman, M., & Stunkard, A. J., Caloric intake and expenditure of obese children. *Journal of Pediatrics,* 1980, *96,* 187–193. Copyright © 1980 by the C. V. Mosby Company. Reprinted by permission of the publisher.

this, for Dr. Solow and his colleagues at Dartmouth (Solow, Siberfarb, & Swift, 1974) were the first to provide a careful description of the psychological sequelae of jejunoileal bypass surgery, the most common surgical treatment for obesity. In this operation, 14 inches of proximal jejunum is anastomosed to four inches of terminal ileum, bypassing the remaining bowel and radically reducing its absorptive surface.

Dr. Solow has described large, and unexpected, improvement in psychosocial functioning of obese persons following jejunoileal bypass surgery when compared to their functioning before surgery. Our own interest has been piqued by an interesting related finding—the benign course of weight loss following surgical treatment of morbid obesity, as compared with the many difficulties during dieting. As we have noted above, untoward responses to dieting afflict many obese persons, and a majority of morbidly obese persons, as illustrated in Table 1.2. To our great surprise, we found a virtual absence of such untoward emotional responses following jejunoileal bypass surgery. A systematic study of this phenomenon (Mills & Stunkard, 1976) revealed that this surgery was followed by a strikingly lower incidence of depression, anxiety, irritability, and preoccupation with food and a strikingly higher incidence of self-confidence and elation than occurred during dieting in patients who had undergone both forms of treatment. Furthermore, we found changes in eating patterns as striking as the differences in emotional responses. Before surgery, most patients reported chaotic patterns of excessive food intake. After surgery, they reported a striking "normalization" of eating patterns: marked decrease in binge eating, excessive snacking, difficulty in stopping eating, and night eating. This decrease in night eating included even the return of appetite for breakfast, a paradox among people who were rapidly losing weight. As striking as the changes in eating patterns was the fact that they occurred without any conscious effort on the part of the patients.

A final aspect of the sequelae of jejunoileal bypass surgery was that decreased food intake and not decreased intestinal absorption was primarily responsible for the large weight losses, losses that averaged 130 pounds in the Mills and Stunkard study. Careful assessment on a metabolic ward permitted Bray and his associates (Bray, 1980; Bray, Dahms, Atkinson, Mena, & Schwartz, 1980) to calculate that no more than 25 percent of the weight loss following jejunoileal bypass is due to malabsorption. Seventy-five percent is due to decreased food intake.

Such profound differences in emotional responses and in eating patterns seem unlikely to have resulted simply from impaired intestinal absorption. They suggest, instead, that the surgery may have brought about major changes in the biology of the organism. But what kind of biological changes could give rise to such profound behavioral changes? The answer may lie in the vicissitudes of the regulation of body weight. A parsimonious explanation is that weight losses following surgery resulted from a resetting of the set point about which body weight is regulated. Such an explanation could account for the relative ease with which obese persons lose weight, for a lowered set point would cause physiological regulation to favor a lowered food intake, rather than oppose it, as is the case during dieting. Persons who eat less in the service of a physiological regulation may find it much easier than those who eat less in opposition to that regulation.

In recent years the severity of the physiological problems associated with jejunoileal bypass surgery and the appearance of new problems for years after surgery persuaded the 1978 Consensus Conference of the National Institutes of Health that continuation of jejunoileal bypass is probably not warranted. The Conference was undoubtedly influenced toward this negative view of jejunoileal bypass by early reports on gastric bypass surgery that indicated that this procedure is followed by far fewer complications. Gastric bypass is a modified Billroth-II operation designed to produce a 60-ml pouch that markedly restricts the amount of food that can be consumed at one time (Mason, Printen, Blommers, & Scott, 1978).

We have recently completed a study of gastric bypass surgery patients, attempting to assess precisely the same issues that we observed among jejunoileal bypass patients—their remarkably benign psychological postoperative course as compared with their experience during reducing diets (Halmi et al., 1980). Much to our surprise, we found that these patients, too, lost weight following surgery with far fewer untoward emotional responses than they had experienced during reducing diets. Table 1.3 shows that over half of the patients reported less intense symptoms after surgery and nearly half reported that these

Table 1.3 Comparison of Untoward Responses after Gastric Bypass with Those during Dieting

	Much Less	Less	Same	More	Much More	Other
Depression	45	9	31	5	5	5
Anxiety	46	15	26	4	4	5
Irritability	49	20	20	4	3	5
Preoccupation with food	48	16	24	3	4	6

symptoms were "much less" intense. Only a very small minority reported that untoward reactions after surgery were greater than those
during their earlier dietary efforts. Furthermore, after jejunoileal
bypass, positive reactions were far more common. Table 1.4 shows that
over half of the patients reported that surgery was followed by a
greater measure of positive emotions than they had experienced during dietary treatment.

This finding, that gastric bypass, as well as jejunoileal bypass, can
produce large weight losses with few untoward emotional responses,
suggests that the two operations produce profound changes in the
biology of the organism. But the operations are quite dissimilar and
their results—emptiness of bowel and small stomach capacity—are
very different. Do these operations produce their similar results by
these very different mechanisms? Perhaps. But the common element
in both appears to be a lowering of body weight set point.

Table 1.4 Comparisons of Positive Responses
after Gastric Bypass with Those during Dieting

	Much More	More	Same	Less	Much Less	Other
Elation	46	6	36	2	4	5
Self-confidence	53	10	24	5	3	6

From Halmi, K. A., Stunkard, A. J., & Mason, E. E. Emotional responses to weight reduction by three
methods: gastric bypass, jejunoileal bypass, and diet. *American Journal of Clinical Nutrition*, 1980, *33*,
446–451. Copyright © 1980 by the American Society of Clinical Nutrition. Reprinted with permission.

Conclusion

This chapter describes the power of the regulation of body weight and
the marked extent to which the body weight of even obese animals is
regulated. This powerful regulation may be responsible for three
common phenomena in the treatment of obesity: dropping out of
treatment, emotional disturbances during dieting, and the regaining
of weight lost during treatment. The regulation of body weight may
also account for the newly described condition of "restrained eating"—
the tendency for habitual dieters to manifest other distinctive behavioral characteristics. It seems likely that both restrained eating and
these problems in treatment occur primarily among persons who are
biologically programmed to be obese, perhaps by an excessive number
of fat cells in their adipose tissue. Perhaps because they are not so

burdened, or perhaps for other reasons, an increasing number of obese people are benefited from a variety of treatments. Psychoanalysis has recently been shown to be relatively effective in weight reduction as well as in decreasing the body-image disparagement of persons afflicted with this disorder. Phenytoin has been able to decrease eating binges in a substantial fraction of bulimics. Recent research has shown that overeating and not underactivity is probably responsible for much of childhood obesity, permitting the development of more effective behavioral treatments. And the newer surgical treatments that seem to be useful for the treatment of morbid obesity may act in a physiological way by affecting the regulation of body weight.

References

Björntorp, P., Carlgren, G., Isaksson, B., Krotkiewski, M., Larsson, B., & Sjöström, L. Effect of an energy-reduced dietary regimen in relation to adipose tissue cellularity in obese women. *American Journal of Clinical Nutrition*, 1975, *28*, 445–452.

Bradfield, R., Paulos, J., & Grossman, H. Energy expenditure and heart rate of obese high school girls. *American Journal of Clinical Nutrition*, 1971, *24*, 1482–1486.

Bray, G. A. Surgical procedures for obesity. In A. J. Stunkard (Ed.), *Obesity*. Philadelphia: Saunders, 1980, pp. 369–387.

Bray, G. A., Dahms, W. T., Atkinson, R. L., Mena, I., & Schwartz, A. Factors controlling food intake. A comparison of dieting and intestinal bypass. *American Journal of Clinical Nutrition*, 1980, *33*, 376–382.

Bruch, H. Obesity in childhood. III. Physiological and psychological aspects of food intake of obese children. *American Journal of Diseases of Children*, 1940, *59*, 739–748.

Bruch, H. Psychological aspects of reducing. *Psychosomatic Medicine*, 1952, *14*, 337–346.

Bullen, B. A., Reed, R. B., & Mayer, J. Physical activity of obese and nonobese adolescent girls appraised by motion picture sampling. *American Journal of Clinical Nutrition*, 1964, *14*, 211–233.

Cahn, A. Growth and caloric intake of heavy and tall children. *Journal of American Dietetic Association*, 1968, *53*, 476–480.

Craighead, L. W., Stunkard, A. J., & O'Brien, R. Behavior therapy and pharmacotherapy of obesity. *Archives of General Psychiatry*, 1981, *38*, 763–768.

Deutsch, F. *On the mysterious leap from the mind to the body: A workshop study on the theory of conversion*. New York: International Universities Press, 1959.

Drenick, E. J., & Johnson, D. Weight reduction by fasting and semi-starvation in morbid obesity: Long-term follow-up. *International Journal of Obesity*, 1978, *2*, 123–132.

Green, R. S., & Rau, J. H. Treatment of compulsive eating disturbances with anticonvulsant medication. *American Journal of Psychiatry*, 1974, *131*, 428–432.

Halmi, K. A., Stunkard, A. J., & Mason, E. E. Emotional responses to weight reduction by three methods: Gastric bypass, jejunoileal bypass, diet. *American Journal of Clinical Nutrition*, 1980, *33*, 446–451.

Hamilton, C. H. Problems of refeeding after starvation in the rat. *Annals of New York Academy of Science*, 1969, *157*, 1004–1017.

Herman, C. P., & Mack, D. Restrained and unrestrained eating. *Journal of Personality*, 1975, *43*, 647–660.

Herman, C. P., & Polivy, J. Anxiety, restraint, and eating behavior. *Journal of Abnormal Psychology*, 1975, *84*, 666–672.

Herman, C. P., & Polivy, J. Restrained eating. In A. J. Stunkard (Ed.), *Obesity*. Philadelphia: Saunders, 1980, pp. 208–225.

Hoebel, R. G., & Teitelbaum, P. Weight regulation in normal and hypothalamic rats. *Journal of Comparative and Physiological Psychology*, 1966, *61*, 189–193.

Keesey, R. E. The regulation of body weight: A set-point analysis. In A. J. Stunkard (Ed.), *Obesity*. Philadelphia: Saunders, 1980, pp. 144–165.

Keys, A., Brozek, J., Henschel, A., Mickelson, D., & Taylor, H. L. *The Biology of Human Starvation*. Minneapolis: University of Minnesota Press, 1950.

Mason, E. E., Printen, K. J., Blommers, T. J., & Scott, D. H. Gastric bypass for obesity after ten years' experience. *International Journal of Obesity*, 1978, *2*, 197–206.

Maxfield, E., & Konishi, F. Patterns of food intake and physical activity in obesity. *Journal of American Dietetic Association*, 1966, *49*, 406–408.

Mills, M. J., & Stunkard, A. J. Behavioral changes following surgery for obesity. *American Journal of Psychiatry*, 1976, *133*, 527–531.

Nisbett, R. E. Hunger, obesity and the ventromedial hypothalamus. *Psychological Review*, 1972, *75*, 433–453.

Rand, C. S. W., & Stunkard, A. J. Psychoanalysis and obesity. *Journal of the American Academy of Psychoanalysis*, 1977, *5*, 459–497.

Rand, C. S. W., & Stunkard, A. J. Obesity and psychoanalysis. *American Journal of Psychiatry*, 1978, *135*, 547–551.

Schachter, S. Some extraordinary facts about humans and rats. *American Psychologist*, 1971, *25*, 129–144.

Schachter, S., Goldman, R., & Gordon, A. Effects of fear, food deprivation, and obesity on eating. *Journal of Personality and Social Psychology*, 1968, *10*, 91–97.

Silverstone, J. T., & Lascelles, B. D. Dieting and depression. *British Journal of Psychiatry*, 1966, *112*, 513–519.

Sims, E. A. H., & Horton, E. S. Endocrine and metabolic adaptation to obesity and starvation. *American Journal of Clinical Nutrition*, 1968, *21*, 1455–1470.

Sjöstrom, L. Fat cells and body weight. In A. J. Stunkard (Ed.), *Obesity*. Philadelphia: Saunders, 1980, pp. 72–100.

Solow, C., Silberfarb, P. M., & Swift, K. Psychosocial effects of intestinal bypass surgery for severe obesity. *New England Journal of Medicine,* 1974, *290,* 300–304.

Stefanic, P. A., Heald, F. P., & Mayer, J. Caloric intake in relation to energy output of obese and nonobese adolescent boys. *American Journal of Clinical Nutrition,* 1959, *7,* 55–62.

Stunkard, A. J. The "dieting depression." *American Journal of Medicine,* 1957, *23,* 77–86.

Stunkard, A. J. Restrained eating: What it is and a new scale to measure it. In L. A. Cioffi (Ed.), *The body weight regulatory system: Normal and disturbed mechanisms.* New York: Raven Press, 1981, pp. 243–251.

Stunkard, A. J., & McLaren-Hume, M. The results of treatment of obesity. A review of the literature and report of a series. *Archives of Internal Medicine,* 1959, *103,* 79–85.

Stunkard, A. J., & Mendelson, M. Obesity and the body image: I. Characteristics of the disturbances in the body image of some obese persons. *American Journal of Psychiatry,* 1967, *123,* 1296–1300.

Stunkard, A. J., & Penick, S. B. Behavior modification in the treatment of obesity: The problem of maintaining weight loss. *Archives of General Psychiatry,* 1979, *36,* 801–806.

Stunkard, A. J., & Pestka, J. The physical activity of obese girls. *American Journal of Diseases of Children,* 1962, *103,* 812–817.

Stunkard, A. J., & Rush, A. J. Dieting and depression reexamined: A critical review of reports of untoward responses during weight reduction for obesity. *Annals of Internal Medicine,* 1974, *81,* 526–533.

Swanson, D. W., & Dinello, F. A. Follow-up of patients starved for obesity. *Psychosomatic Medicine,* 1970, *32,* 209–214.

Waxman, M., & Stunkard, A. J. Caloric intake and expenditure of obese children. *Journal of Pediatrics,* 1980, *96,* 187–193.

Weissenburger, J., Rush, A. J., Giles, D. E., Kumetz, N., & Stunkard, A. J. Determinants of weight change in depressed patients. *Journal of Consulting and Clinical Psychology,* in press.

Wermuth, B. M., Davis, K. L., Hollister, L. E., & Stunkard, A. J. Phenytoin treatment of the binge-eating syndrome. *American Journal of Psychiatry,* 1977, *134,* 1249–1253.

Wilkinson, P. W., Parklin, J. M., Pearloom, G., Strong, M., & Sykes, P. Energy intake and physical activity in obese children. *British Medical Journal,* 1977, *1,* 756.

Wirtshafter, D., & Davis, J. D. Set points, settling points and the control of body weight. *Physiology and Behavior,* 1977, *19,* 75–78.

2
Surgical Treatment of Obesity

Charles Solow

Surgical treatment of obesity is of interest from two standpoints: For the clinician, surgery is the only therapeutic approach, at present, to achieve substantial and lasting weight loss in the severely obese (Leon, 1979; Van Itallie, 1980). As a treatment modality, it is very much with us. In 1978 it was estimated that over 60,000 surgical procedures for obesity had been performed in this country (Yates, 1980). To paraphrase a surgeon (Buckwald, 1979) who has performed and carefully studied the results of over 1000 such operations, the surgical approach to obesity is similar to attempting to repair one's TV set with a monkey wrench. (He puts it that "surgical treatment is an approximation to rational therapy.") Surgery carries an appreciable mortality and morbidity; there is general agreement that it should be considered only for massive or "morbid" obesity (weight in excess of 100 percent or 100 pounds over desirable weight as determined by standard tables).

For the scholar, surgical amelioration of obesity offers unique opportunities to learn about pathogenetic mechanisms in obesity.

This review first describes the various surgical techniques that are utilized, then summarizes clinical observations of the psychosocial consequences of surgically induced weight loss, and finally will consider some studies deriving from surgical treatment which hold promise of a better understanding of the psychobiology of obesity.

Surgical Techniques

Surgical procedures in widespread use fall into two categories: Those which involve bypassing much of the intestinal tract and those which aim at reduction of gastric capacity and emptying.

The first intestinal shunt to be tried was a jejunocolic bypass in which the ileum was totally excluded (Payne, DeWind, & Commons, 1963). This procedure was soon rejected because of an unacceptable incidence of intractable diarrhea, nutritional and electrolyte depletion, and liver damage. Payne introduced the end-to-side jejunoileal bypass in the late 1950s (Payne & DeWind, 1969); the end-to-end jejunoileal bypass was initiated in the early 1960s (Salmon, 1971; Scott, Dean, Shull, & Gluck, 1977). Both variations of jejunoileal bypass exclude about 90 percent of the small intestine (i.e., all but 50 cm) from the alimentary stream. The defunctionalized bowel is not removed, and the procedure can be reversed. Each variation has its advocates; many clinicians view them as roughly equivalent in value.

Weight loss, which levels off during the second postoperative year, is substantial (about 45 kg or 35 percent of initial weight, on the average) and lasting. This weight loss was initially thought to be the result of malabsorption, but it has been clearly demonstrated that the mechanism is more complex. Only one-third of weight reduction is due to malabsorption; two-thirds is a reflection of reduced food intake (Bray, Dahms, Atkinson, Rodin, Taylor, Frame, & Schwartz, 1979; Condon, Janes, Wise, & Alpers, 1978; Robinson, Folstein, & McHugh, 1979). Ingested calories drop from preoperative levels of over 6000 per day to about 2000 calories during the first six months after surgery. Somatic benefits include a reduction in blood pressure, improved exercise tolerance and cardiorespiratory function, alleviation of musculoskeletal problems aggravated by obesity (e.g., low back pain), and improvement in venous stasis difficulties in the legs. Glucose tolerance improves, and serum cholesterol and triglycerides are consistently lowered.

Mortality rates reported by experienced surgeons are about 3 percent (*Medical Letter*, 1978). Serious side effects and complications are frequent enough to render the justifiability of jejunoileal shunting problematic (Halverson, 1980). Diarrhea, which occurs with almost all patients for a time after surgery, can be a persistent and severe problem for some. Associated difficulties include persistent electrolyte depletion, protein malnutrition, and debilitating fatigue. Cholelithiasis occurs with increased frequency following surgery. Foul-smelling stools and flatus become socially handicapping for some patients. Abdominal bloating is common, and in its more severe form can progress to bypass enteritis, proctitis, and pseudo-obstructive megacolon, all apparently the result of bacterial overgrowth in the defunctionalized bowel. Hepatic failure—related to protein malnutrition and/or to bacterial overgrowth—has caused 1 to 2 percent of the deaths and is an indication for shunt reversal (reanastomosis). Polyarthritis/

arthralgia is yet another complication seemingly related to bacterial overgrowth in the bypassed bowel. Oxalate kidney stones occur in up to 25 percent of cases and reflect increased absorption of dietary oxalate. Focal interstitial nephritis and bone changes are two recently described late complications of this surgery.

This is a long and rather grim list. Hence, it is all the more striking that all series report about a 90 percent patient acceptance rate: most patients would choose to have the operation if again faced with the decision (Quaade, 1979; Yates, 1980). Some patients resist, literally to the death, advice to have the bypass taken down because of complications. This tells us something about the suffering that these patients experience because of morbid obesity and how intensely averse they are to returning to their prior obese state. (Most will regain every bit of lost weight following reanastomosis, unless the intestinal bypass is replaced by a gastric bypass.)

Gastric reduction procedures originated in 1966 when Mason began performing gastric bypasses (Mason, Printen, Blommers, Lewis, & Scott, 1980). A number of modifications have been made upon Mason's original technique; more recently reinforced gastroplasty (Gomez, 1980) and gastric partitioning (Pace, Martin, Tetrick, Fabri, & Carey, 1979) have been introduced. All of these techniques aim at the creation of a small, 50 cc gastric pouch with a stomal egress no larger than 12 mm. This results in rapid filling and slowed emptying of the stomach, and this in turn enhances satiety. Weight loss, which is roughly equivalent to that achieved by intestinal bypass, is clearly a consequence of reduction in food intake. Because nutrients pass through most, if not all, of the gastrointestinal tract, and there is no large segment of defunctionalized bowel, most of the severe complications of intestinal shunting are avoided. Thus, diarrhea, electrolyte depletion, and severe malnutrition, kidney stones, hepatic damage, accelerated cholelithiasis, arthritis, nephritis, and enteritis are not encountered. Expected complications (stomal ulceration, anastomotic leaks, dumping, stomal obstruction) have either been infrequent or relatively easily managed. Most reoperation in the case of the gastric procedure has been to revise the pouch or stoma after inadequate weight loss; in contrast, most reoperation in the case of intestinal shunts has been for reanastomosis because of unacceptable complications.

Intestinal bypass procedures have been performed over a longer span of time and by many more surgeons than the gastric procedures. Hence, more is known about the long-range effects of intestinal shunting.

Because the attendant morbidity with gastric reduction procedures is distinctly less severe and the benefits roughly equivalent, there
is a growing trend to abandon jejunoileal bypass operations in favor of
gastric procedures (Alden, 1977; Baddely, 1979; Buckwalter, 1980;
Griffin, Young, & Stevenson, 1977; Linner, 1980; MacLean, Rochon,
Munro, Watson, & Shizgal, 1980; Petier, Hemreck, Moffat, Hardin, &
Jewell, 1979; Quaade, 1979). Many intestinal shunts have been converted to gastric bypasses, with maintenance of weight loss. Within
gastric surgery, the trend is away from bypass and toward simpler
techniques, such as gastric stapling (partitioning), which avoids the
necessity for anastomosis.

Jaw wiring (or maxillomandibular fixation), though used successfully to achieve substantial weight loss, is invariably followed by weight
regain after the wires are cut (Kark, 1980). Truncal vagotomy is reported to result in weight loss, but it is too early for even a tentative
judgment of the value of this procedure (Kral, 1980).

Psychosocial Consequences

Almost all the observations of psychosocial effects of surgically induced
weight loss have concerned jejunoileal bypass. In the early years there
was concern that since this treatment "removed" the "symptom" of
obesity without resolving any of the putative underlying psychological
conflicts, surgery would often have adverse psychological sequelae.
That this has not proven to be the case constitutes a challenge to this
simplistic psychogenic concept of obesity (Solow, Silberfarb, & Swift,
1974). Most studies note a generally, often impressively favorable
psychosocial outcome (Danish Obesity Project, 1979; Castelnuovo-
Tedesco, 1980; Kuldau & Rand, 1980b; Leon, Eckert, Teed, & Buckwald, 1979; Salzstein & Gutmann, 1980; Solow, Silberfarb, & Swift,
1978). With weight loss, patients report improvement in activity levels
(social and physical), mood, self-esteem, and interpersonal and voca-
tional effectiveness. More normal satiety mechanisms and eating behavior often emerge. With many patients a self-reinforcing sense of
entrapment, ineffectiveness, and failure is replaced by hope and
awareness of increased opportunity. There seems to be decreased
reliance upon denial as a coping mechanism; patients are more "in
touch with" and expressive of their feelings and are more likely to
recognize and acknowledge unpleasant circumstances. This change
was described in different ways. Thus, one study (Dano & Hahn-

Pederson, 1977) noted a "normalization" of temper postoperatively; that is, preoperatively the patients were "abnormally" good tempered. Body image, an important element in self-esteem, consistently changes from self-disparagement and self-consciousness to realistic self-acceptance. Thus, "mirror avoidance" often ends, and more patients venture forth in bathing suits.

As self-esteem and self-confidence improve, passivity diminishes, self-assertiveness increases, and a greater sense of autonomy and independence develops. Not surprisingly these changes often result in interpersonal reappraisals and realignments, which are sometimes quite painful. Marital conflict and breakup are not uncommon sequelae to surgery. As noted by one study (Neill, Marshall, & Yale, 1978), massive obesity seems to have acted as a stabilizing factor in some rather brittle, unsatisfying marriages. It would appear that most marriages are either unchanged or improved by weight loss after surgery (Solow et al., 1978; Kuldau & Rand, 1980b).

Untoward affective responses, indeed, frank psychiatric illnesses, do occur postoperatively. These psychological problems often are reactions to somatic complications, are continuing events in a pattern antedating surgery, or are responses to adventitious environmental events, rather than consequences of weight loss (Solow, 1977; Kuldau & Rand, 1980a). Such untoward affective states seem generally less frequent after weight loss than preoperatively. In a small number of patients, psychosocial problems arise from the challenge presented to the patient's coping abilities by the implications of weight loss; these difficulties constitute illness of increased opportunity. Emotional turmoil in a patient enabled by weight loss to return to school may be viewed in this light. There is a growing consensus that such psychological difficulties do not mean that surgery is unwarranted, or that such patients should be "screened out" psychiatrically, or that for these patients obesity provides an obligatory defense. Rather, it seems clear that psychiatric/psychological consultation must be readily available to patients undergoing surgery for obesity. Given appropriate assistance, patients will often come through their emotional difficulties with more flexible and adaptive modes of coping (Solow et al., 1978).

Since the psychological constellation associated with obesity (inactivity, low self-esteem, passivity, vulnerability to depression, body-image disparagement) is reversible to a surprising degree, these characteristics appear to be as much the result as they are the cause of obesity.

The only justifiable psychiatric grounds for ruling out or delaying surgery would seem to be: (1) active psychosis, (2) continuing strong ambivalence about having the surgery, (3) demonstrated unreliability in adhering to medical programs, and (4) alcoholism (Kuldau & Rand, 1980b; Solow, 1977).

Further Studies of Psychobiology

One line of inquiry concerning the effects of surgery has made a start in elucidating the psychobiological determinants of obesity. Stunkard and co-workers have suggested that comparing the emotional status of patients while losing weight after surgery to their condition just before surgery results in an underestimation of the salutory effects of surgical intervention. They have assessed the emotional status of patients while losing weight postoperatively, after both jejunoileal bypass (Mills & Stunkard, 1976) and gastric bypass (Halmi, Stunkard, & Mason, 1980), and compared it retrospectively to the same patient's past experience while attempting to lose weight by dieting.

It has been noted that the morbidly obese frequently develop dysphoric states of depression, anxiety, irritability, and preoccupation with thoughts of food when dieting is attempted. So it was with these patients. Surgically induced weight loss was accompanied by far less dysphoria than was dieting. Indeed, the patients frequently reported unprecedented feelings of elation and self-confidence while losing weight postoperatively. Furthermore, normalization of eating behavior was noted to occur after jejunoileal bypass (decreased frequency of eating binges, less night eating, less snacking, reduced craving for sweets, decreased food consumption in general, fewer meals, increased frequency of breakfast consumption).

The changes that were induced by surgery were, in Stunkard's view, so profound as to suggest a change in the biology of the obese person. The findings are felt to support the concept of obesity as an alteration of the set point about which body weight is regulated.

The results of these studies are confirmed and extended by Bray and co-workers. They compared the effects of weight loss by dieting and that following jejunoileal bypass in a prospective fashion (Bray et al., 1979). Again, patients experienced less depression, anger, and preoccupation with food and had more positive affects after surgery than with dieting. Again, there was a normalization of eating behavior and also of taste perception during weight loss following surgery, but not after dieting. Concomitant biochemical assays were carried out from which emerged a consistent change in the internal milieu that might represent a change in the set point about which body weight is regulated. After jejunoileal bypass, but not after dieting, there was a drop in basal and post-meal insulin, a rise in basal glycerol, a decrease in post-meal glucose, and increases in postprandial pancreatic polypeptide and postprandial enteroglucagon.

Conclusion

In the near future there will probably be further ingenious refinements of gastric-reduction surgery and further study of new complex techniques such as biliopancreatic bypass (Scoparino, Gianetta, Civalleri, Bonalumi, & Bachi, 1980). Ultimately, better understanding of the basic psychobiology of obesity should allow the surgeon to turn to other matters while less invasive techniques are employed to alter the regulation of weight.

References

Alden, J. F. Gastric and jejunoileal bypass. A comparison in the treatment of morbid obesity. *Archives of Surgery,* 1977, *112,* 799–806.

Baddely, R. M. The management of gross refractory obesity by jejunoileal bypass. *British Journal of Surgery,* 1979, *66,* 525–532.

Bray, G. A., Dahms, W. T., Atkinson, R. L., Rodin, J., Taylor, I., Frame, C., & Schwartz, A. Metabolic and behavioral differences between dieting and intestinal bypass. *Hormone and Metabolic Research,* 1979, *11,* 648–654.

Buckwald, H. Foreword. Symposium on morbid obesity. *Surgical Clinics of North America,* 1979, *59,* 961–962.

Buckwalter, J. A. Morbid obesity: Good and poor results of jejunoileal and gastric bypass. *American Journal of Clinical Nutrition,* 1980, *33,* 476–480.

Castelnuovo-Tedesco, P. Jejunoileal bypass for superobesity: A psychiatric assessment. *Advances in Psychosomatic Medicine,* 1980, *10,* 196–206.

Condon, S. C., Janes, N. J., Wise, L., & Alpers, D. H. Role of calorie intake in the weight loss after jejunoileal bypass for obesity. *Gastroenterology,* 1978, *74,* 34–37.

Danish Obesity Project, The. Randomized trial of jejunoileal bypass versus medical treatment in morbid obesity. *Lancet,* 1979, *ii,* 1255–1257.

Dano, P., & Hahn-Pederson, J. Improvement in quality of life following jejunoileal bypass surgery for obesity. *Scandinavian Journal of Gastroenterology,* 1977, *12,* 769–774.

Gomez, C. A. Gastroplasty in the surgical treatment of morbid obesity. *American Journal of Clinical Nutrition,* 1980, *33,* 406–415.

Griffin, W. O., Young, V. L., & Stevenson, C. C. A prospective comparison of gastric and jejunoileal bypass procedures for morbid obesity. *Annals of Surgery*, 1977, *186*, 500–509.

Halmi, K. A., Stunkard, A. J., & Mason, E. E. Emotional responses to weight reduction by three methods: gastric bypass, jejunoileal bypass, diet. *American Journal of Clinical Nutrition*, 1980, *33*, 446–451.

Halverson, J. D. Obesity surgery in perspective. *Surgery*, 1980, *87*, 119–127.

Kark, A. E. Jaw wiring. *American Journal of Clinical Nutrition*, 1980, *33*, 420–424.

Kral, J. G. Effects of truncal vagotomy on body weight and hyperinsulinemia in morbid obesity. *American Journal of Clinical Nutrition*, 1980, *33*, 416–419.

Kuldau, J. M., & Rand, C. S. W. Negative psychiatric sequelae to jejunoileal bypass are often not correlated with operative results. *American Journal of Clinical Nutrition*, 1980, *33*, 502–503.(a)

Kuldau, J. M., & Rand, C. S. W. Jejunoileal bypass: General and psychiatric outcome after one year. *Psychosomatics*, 1980, *21*, 534–539.(b)

Leon, G. R. Personality and morbid obesity. Implications for dietary management through behavior modification. *Surgical Clinics of North America*, 1979, *59*, 1007–1015.

Leon, G. R., Eckert, E. D., Teed, D., & Buckwald, H. Changes in body image and other psychological factors after intestinal bypass surgery for massive obesity. *Journal of Behavioral Medicine*, 1979, *2*, 39–55.

Linner, J. H. A summary of 24 years' experience with surgery for morbid obesity. *American Journal of Clinical Nutrition*, 1980, *33*, 504–505.

MacLean, L. D., Rochon, G., Munro, M., Watson, K. E. L., & Shizgal, H. M. Intestinal bypass for morbid obesity: A consecutive personal experience. *Canadian Journal of Surgery*, 1980, *23*, 54–59.

Mason, E. E., Printen, K. J., Blommers, T. J., Lewis, J. W., & Scott, D. H. Gastric bypass in morbid obesity. *American Journal of Clinical Nutrition*, 1980, *33*, 395–405.

Medical Letter on Drugs and Therapeutics, The. Bypass operations for obesity. 1978, *20*, 33–35.

Mills, M. J., & Stunkard, A. J. Behavioral changes following surgery for obesity. *American Journal of Psychiatry*, 1976, *133*, 527–531.

Neill, J. R., Marshall, A. R., & Yale, C. E. Marital changes after intestinal bypass surgery. *Journal of the American Medical Association*, 1978, *240*, 447–450.

Pace, W. G., Martin, E. W., Jr., Tetrick, T., Fabri, P. J., & Carey, L. C. Gastric partitioning for morbid obesity. *Annals of Surgery*, 1979, *190*, 392–400.

Payne, J. H., & DeWind, L. T. Surgical treatment of obesity. *American Journal of Surgery*, 1969, *118*, 141–147.

Payne, J. H., DeWind, L. T., & Commons, R. R. Metabolic observations on patients with jejunocolic shunt. *American Journal of Surgery*, 1963, *106*, 273–289.

Petier, G., Hemreck, A. S., Moffat, R. E., Hardin, C. A., & Jewell, W. R. Complications following gastric bypass procedures for morbid obesity. *Surgery*, 1979, *86*, 648–654.

Quaade, F. Jejunoileal bypass for morbid obesity. A bibliographic study and a randomized clinical trial. *Surgical Clinics of North America*, 1979, *59*, 1055–1069.

Robinson, R. G., Folstein, M. F., & McHugh, P. R. Reduced caloric intake following small bowel bypass surgery; a systematic study of possible causes. *Psychological Medicine*, 1979, *9*, 37–53.

Salmon, P. A. The results of small intestine bypass operations for the treatment of obesity. *Surgery, Gynecology and Obstetrics*, 1971, *132*, 965–979.

Salzstein, E. C., & Gutmann, M. D. Gastric bypass for morbid obesity. Preoperative and postoperative psychological evaluation of patients. *Archives of Surgery*, 1980, *115*, 21–28.

Scoparino, N., Gianetta, E., Civalleri, D., Bonalumi, U., & Bachi, V. Two years of clinical experience with biliopancreatic bypass for obesity. *American Journal of Clinical Nutrition*, 1980, *33*, 506–514.

Scott, H. W., Jr., Dean, R. H., Shull, H. J., & Gluck, F. Results of jejunoileal bypass in two hundred patients with morbid obesity. *Surgery, Gynecology, and Obstetrics*, 1977, *145*, 661–673.

Solow, C. Psychosocial aspects of intestinal bypass surgery for massive obesity: Current status. *American Journal of Clinical Nutrition*, 1977, *30*, 103–108.

Solow, C., Silberfarb, P. M., & Swift, K. Psychosocial effects of intestinal bypass surgery for severe obesity. *New England Journal of Medicine*, 1974, *290*, 300–304.

Solow, C., Silberfarb, P. M., & Swift, K. Psychological and behavioral consequences of intestinal bypass. In G. A. Bray (Ed.), *Recent advances in obesity research*, Vol. II. London: Newman Publications, 1978.

Van Itallie, T. B. "Morbid" obesity: A hazardous disorder that resists conservative treatment. *American Journal of Clinical Nutrition*, 1980, *33*, 358–363.

Yates, B. T. Survey comparison of success, morbidity, mortality, fees and psychological benefits and costs of 3,146 patients receiving jejunoileal or gastric bypass. *American Journal of Clinical Nutrition*, 1980, *33*, 518–522.

3

Obesity: Behavioral Treatments for a Serious, Prevalent, and Refractory Problem

Kelly D. Brownell

Obesity is one of the most puzzling disorders of modern times. It has been long recognized that the obese state is difficult for many people to avoid. William Beaumont described this problem in 1883:

> In the present state of civilized society with the provocation of the culinary art, and the incentive of highly seasoned foods, brandy, and wine, the temptation to excess in the indulgences of the table are rather too strong to be resisted by poor human nature [Beaumont, 1959, p. 4].

The current public view of obesity is not nearly so charitable. The obese person is viewed as a self-indulgent, weak-willed, and lazy individual who is gratified only by eating to excess. In contrast, the scientific community views obesity as a complex phenomenon with multiple origins (Bray, 1976; Stunkard, 1980). The study of obesity and its treatment spans many disciplines, including physiology, psychology, psychiatry, nutrition, metabolism, sociology, and anthropology.

The Consequences of Obesity

Prevalence

Obesity is the number one nutrition problem in the United States (U.S. Senate, 1977). Between 15 and 30 percent of adult Americans are obese (Bray, 1979; Van Itallie, 1979). The prevalence is even higher with advancing age, with decreasing socioeconomic status, and in some ethnic groups (Stunkard, 1975). The prevalence of obesity is alarming even in children. Between 10 and 15 percent of young children are obese, and by adolescence the figure increases to 30 percent (Garn & Clark, 1976). Many adults feel the obese child will "grow out of it." They await an unlikely event. Fully 80 percent of overweight children become overweight adults (Abraham & Nordsieck, 1960). Stunkard and Burt (1967) estimated that if an obese child has not slimmed down by the end of adolescence, the odds against his or her doing so as an adult are 28 to 1.

The Medical and Psychological Hazards of Obesity

It is clear that obesity afflicts a large percentage of the population. This fact has important implications for public health, because obesity is associated with many serious problems, both medical and psychological. Insulin insensitivity and diabetes mellitus are more common among obese persons (Drash, 1973; Gordon, Castelli, Hjortland, Kannel, & Dawber, 1977). Impaired pulmonary function is likely in obese persons, and renal problems have been noted in massively obese persons (Bray, 1976; Van Itallie, 1979). Obesity is also associated with surgical risk, greater risk with anesthesia, and complications during pregnancy (Bray, 1976).

The most important medical hazard of obesity lies in its association with coronary heart disease (Gordon & Kannel, 1973) (Figure 3.1). Results from the Framingham Study indicate that obesity influences risk for heart disease, probably through its association with hyperlipidemia, hypertension, and carbohydrate intolerance (Gordon & Kannel, 1973). Relative weight is positively correlated with elevated levels of low-density lipoprotein cholesterol (Kannel, Gordon, & Castelli, 1979), and hypertension is more common among obese persons than among thin persons (Chiang, Perlman, & Epstein, 1969; Kannel & Gordon, 1979) (Figure 3.2). Some researchers claim that obesity is not a coronary risk factor independent of its effects on blood lipids and blood pressure (Mann, 1974), but others present data that indicate that such an independent effect does exist (Kannel & Gordon, 1979). Gordon and Kannel (1973) note that, "Obesity is probably the most common metabolic disorder affecting mankind. It is a serious condition adversely affecting several organ systems, causing decades of disability and contributing to premature death" (p. 88).

The psychological and social hazards of obesity may be as serious

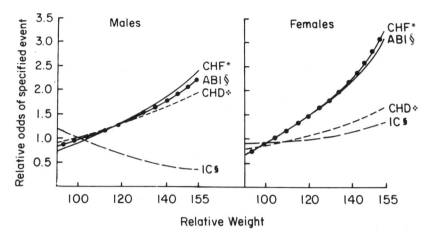

Figure 3.1. Relative risk of cardiovascular events according to relative weight for men and women in a 16-year follow-up of the Framingham Study. Relative weight is the ratio of actual weight to ideal weight multiplied by 100.

From Gordon, T., & Kannel, W. B. The effects of overweight on cardiovascular disease. *Geriatrics*, 1973, *28*, 80–88. Copyright © 1973 by Modern Medicine Publications, Inc., Harcourt Brace Jovanovich Publications. Reprinted by permission of the author and the publisher.

as the medical hazards. The perils of obesity are not apparent in some obese persons, but in many, the long-term consequences of excess weight can be far-ranging, disabling, and permanent (Dwyer & Mayer, 1975; Stunkard, 1976; Stunkard & Mendelson, 1967).

There is little doubt that obesity is a social handicap (Brownell & Stunkard, 1978; Dwyer & Mayer, 1975). The bias against obesity is surprising in both its strength and its early development. In one study, boys ages six to ten assigned characteristics to silhouettes of fat, thin, and muscular boys (Staffieri, 1967). Responses to the muscular silhouette were positive, whereas the fat body type evoked objectionable labels like lazy, sloppy, cheat, forgetful, naughty, dirty, ugly, and stupid. Two other studies had children and adults rate six line drawings depicting a normal child, a child with a brace on one leg with

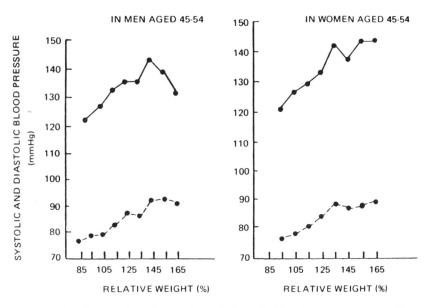

Figure 3.2. Regression of systolic and diastolic blood pressure on relative weight for men and women ages 45 to 54 in the Framingham Study. Relative weight is the ratio of actual weight to ideal weight multiplied by 100.

From Kannel, W. B., & Gordon, T. Physiological and medical concomitants of obesity: The Framingham Study. In G. A. Bray (Ed.), *Obesity in America,* Washington, D.C.: U.S. Department of Health, Education and Welfare, NIH Publication No. 79-359, 1979. Reprinted by permission of the author.

crutches, a child sitting in a wheelchair with a blanket covering both legs, a child with one hand missing, a child with a facial disfigurement, and a grossly overweight child (Maddox, Back, & Liederman, 1968; Richardson, Hastorf, Goodman, & Dornbush, 1961). The overweight child was consistently rated as the least likable.

The social stigma of obesity affects the life of nearly every obese person. Obese persons not only suffer from the social and sometimes physical disability of their excess weight, but they are blamed for their condition. Unlike persons with other physical disabilities, obese people are labeled with terms that connote responsibility (self-indulgent, gluttonous, etc.).

The most common psychological concomitant of obesity is body-image disparagement (Stunkard & Mendelson, 1967). Body image refers to a person's impression of his or her physical appearance and to the associated feelings. Body image in obese persons is characterized by the feeling that one's body is grotesque and detestable and that others view it with contempt and hostility (Stunkard & Mendelson, 1967). This disturbance can lead to intense self-consciousness and to the notion that the world views overweight people with disdain. Consequently, persons with body-image disparagement tend to be withdrawn, shy, and socially immature.

An important psychological hazard of obesity lies in its remedy. Dieting is clearly related to untoward emotional symptoms (Stunkard & Rush, 1974). This is an important problem because many obese persons are "career dieters" who attempt countless methods to reduce. One retrospective study of emotional reactions during dieting in 100 obese persons found that 54 percent experienced emotional symptoms at least once; 21 percent experienced nervousness, 21 percent weakness, 8 percent irritability, 5 percent fatigue, and 4 percent nausea (Stunkard, 1957). Another report found that 50 percent of obese persons experienced the onset or intensification of depression when dieting (Silverstone & Lascelles, 1966). Stunkard (1976) concluded that "Most forms of dieting carry with them a high likelihood of emotional disturbance" (p. 88).

Behavior Therapy: Program Components

Against the backdrop of discouraging results from most treatments, behavior therapy emerged with much fanfare. In 1967 Stuart applied the principles of behavior therapy to the treatment of eight subjects. Figure 3.3, showing losses for four of Stuart's subjects, indicates the results that spawned a decade of research on the behavioral treatment of obesity. By the mid-1970s more than 75 articles had appeared on this approach, and by 1980, this figure more than doubled. The remainder of this chapter will describe the behavior therapy program, its effectiveness, and promising new developments in treatment.

The behavior therapy program outlined here is that used in my research at the University of Pennsylvania (Brownell, 1979; 1980). The program is presented in abbreviated form. It is similar to other behavior therapy programs, each of which owe a great debt to Stuart's original work (1967). Detailed material on the behavioral approach has been published by Ferguson (1975), Jeffrey and Katz (1977), Jordan, Levitz, and Kimbrell (1977), Mahoney and Mahoney (1976), Stuart (1978), and Stuart and Davis (1972).

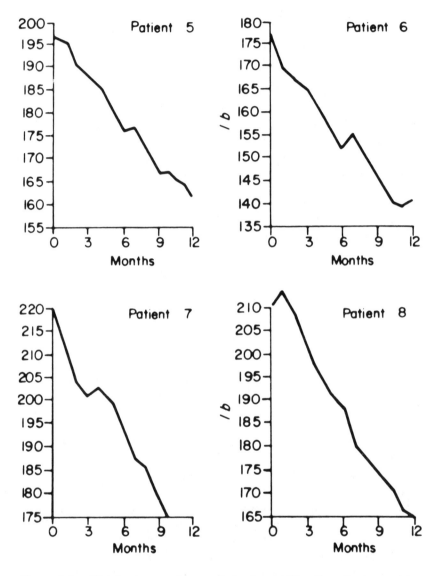

Figure 3.3. Weight changes in pounds for four of Stuart's patients receiving behavior therapy.

Reprinted with permission from *Behaviour Research and Therapy,* Vol. 5, Stuart, R. B., Behavioral control of overeating. Copyright © 1967, Pergamon Press, Ltd.

Behavior therapy began long before its principles were applied to the treatment of obesity. It is a fundamental departure from the psychodynamic and medical models of treatment (Bandura, 1969), and its roots can be traced to the work of Wolpe (1958) in South Africa, Eysenck (1959) in England, and Skinner (1953) in the United States (Wilson & O'Leary, 1980). The core characteristics of behavior therapy are presented in Table 3.1, adapted from Wilson and O'Leary (1980).

Table 3.1. Core Characteristics of Behavior Therapy

---

1. Most abnormal behavior is acquired and maintained according to the same principles as normal behavior.
2. Most abnormal behavior can be modified through the application of social learning principles.
3. Assessment is continuous and focuses on current determinants of behavior.
4. A person is best described by what he or she thinks, feels, and does in specific life situations.
5. Treatment is derived from the theory and experimental findings of scientific psychology, particularly social learning principles.
6. Treatment methods are precisely specified, replicable, and objectively evaluated.
7. Innovative research strategies have been developed to evaluate the effects of specific therapeutic techniques on particular problems.
8. Treatment outcome is evaluated in terms of initial induction of behavior change, its generalization to the real-life setting, and its maintenance over time.
9. Treatment strategies are individually tailored to different problems in different individuals.
10. Extensive use is made of psychological assistants such as parents and teachers to modify problem behavior in the real-life settings where it occurs.
11. Behavior therapy is broadly applicable to a full range of clinical disorders and educational problems.
12. Behavior therapy is a humanistic approach in which treatment goals and methods are mutually contracted, rather than arbitrarily imposed.

From Wilson, G. T., & O'Leary, K. D. *Principles of behavior therapy.* Englewood Cliffs, N.J.: Prentice-Hall, 1980, p. 25. Copyright © 1980 by Prentice-Hall, Inc. Reprinted by permission of the author and the publisher.

The Behavioral Scheme for Treatment

The premise underlying behavior therapy for obesity is that eating *habits* must change for long-term weight loss to occur. The focus in this approach is on *how* rather than *what* the obese person eats. This assumes not that obese and lean people differ in their eating habits, but that changes in habits will allow the obese person to lose weight and keep it off.

The popular notion of the behavioral approach is that of a simplistic program in which the obese person is prescribed a number of "tricks." As is evident in the next sections, a comprehensive behavioral program devotes considerable attention to attitudes and feelings of the obese person, to the social setting in which weight loss occurs, and to interactions among the obese person and the family. In addition, physical activity is gaining more and more emphasis in behavioral programs, a topic discussed later.

Figure 3.4 presents a schematic diagram of the behavioral program. Assessment of the individual's eating and exercise patterns is the first step. This information is then used to form a diagnostic impression of promising areas for intervention. It becomes clear at this point that individuals show great variation in their eating life-styles. For example, one person may consume 95 percent of the day's calories between dinnertime and bedtime and may have no difficulty controlling intake away from home. Another may consume the day's calories in ten separate eating episodes, and location may be unimportant. Techniques are then developed to alter the "ABCs" of behavior: the

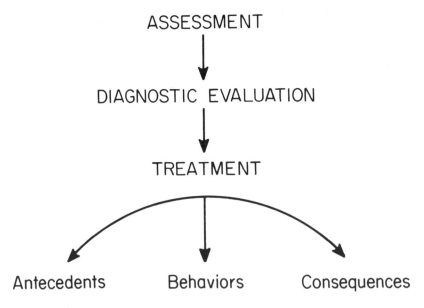

Figure 3.4. A schematic diagram of the behavioral approach to the analysis and treatment of obesity.

antecedents (events that prompt eating), the *behavior* itself (eating topography), and the *consequences* (events that follow eating).

The behavior therapy program is typically administered in groups of eight to 12 patients. There is some evidence that group therapy is more effective than individual therapy (Kingsley & Wilson, 1977), perhaps because of the social support available among the group members. Our program is administered in 16 weekly sessions, with booster sessions occurring every other month for the year following treatment. In our earlier programs, booster sessions were held more frequently, but experimental evidence suggests this does not improve treatment results (Ashby & Wilson, 1977; Craighead, Stunkard, & O'Brien, 1980; Kingsley & Wilson, 1977; Wilson & Brownell, 1978). Each session lasts approximately 1½ hours. Each patient is weighed privately before each session. The group meetings consist of didactic presentation of the week's material and discussion among group members. A deposit-refund procedure is used to reduce attrition from treatment. Patients deposit money (irrespective of whether a treatment fee is charged), which is returned for attendance. The presence or absence of such a deposit appears more important than the amount, and it may be a powerful means of keeping patients in treatment (Wilson & Brownell, 1980).

Self-monitoring

Self-monitoring (recording one's behavior) is common to all behavior therapy programs and is usually identified by patients as the program's most important component. Born as an assessment method, self-monitoring has played a useful role as an active therapeutic procedure. Early behavior therapy programs used self-monitoring to gather data on an individual's eating habits, but it was discovered quickly that the act of recording one's own behavior can alter the behavior under inspection.

Two self-monitoring forms are used in my program: a Diet Diary record of food intake, and a Daily Log measure of habit change (Brownell, 1980). The Diet Diary is a handy, pocket-sized booklet in which 30 pages are available for patients to record a day's eating on each page. Patients begin keeping the Diet Diary in the first week of treatment and record all food eaten and the calorie contents of the food. As the patients become proficient, the Diet Diary is expanded to include more information on eating patterns, including times, locations, other people present, feelings, and other activities. Figure 3.5 is one day's entry for the Diet Diary.

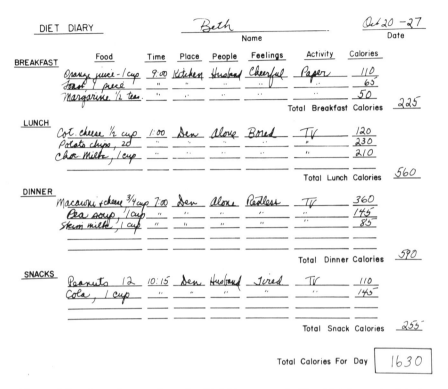

Figure 3.5. Sample entry from the Diet Diary record of food intake and related behavior.

The Diet Diary serves several useful clinical functions. First, it provides information for the therapist to analyze each individual's eating patterns. Second, it can increase self-awareness in the patient; automatic eating patterns that may be given little thought become more evident when recorded. The Diet Diary presented in Figure 3.5, for example, may aid this patient in realizing that most food is eaten while she watches television. Third, many patients report eating less if they know the food will appear in the Diary. Fourth, the Diary educates patients about calories—the final arbiter of weight change.

The second self-monitoring record, the Daily Log, is used as an index of whether patients are following the prescribed treatment regimen. The Daily Log lists the behaviors prescribed for a given week, and the patient rates the degree to which the behaviors are carried out. Figure 3.6 is a sample Daily Log, which covers the behaviors prescribed for that week as well as two categories that are measured throughout the program—keeping the Diet Diary and restricting caloric intake.

DIETER'S DAILY LOG - WEEK ___7___

POINTS: ALL OF THE TIME = 5 POINTS
  MOST OF THE TIME = 3 POINTS
  SOME OF THE TIME = 1 POINT
  NOT AT ALL   = 0 POINTS

Beth
NAME

			DAY				
	Mon.	Tues.	Wed.	Thurs.	Fri.	Sat.	Sun.
1. DID I FILL OUT THE DIET DIARY AFTER EATING?	5	5	3	5	3	5	5
2. Did I keep food out of sight?	5	3	3	1	1	5	3
3. Did I avoid being a food dispenser?	5	5	5	5	5	5	5
4. Did I remove serving dishes after serving?	3	0	5	5	5	3	5
5. Did I use smaller utensils?	3	0	5	5	5	3	5
6. Did I leave the table after eating?	5	0	5	5	5	3	5
HOW MANY CALORIES DID I HAVE TODAY? FOR WOMEN 1000-1200 = 5 POINTS 1200-1500 = 3 POINTS 1500-1700 = 1 POINT ABOVE 1700 = 0 POINTS FOR MEN 1200-1500 = 5 POINTS 1500-1800 = 3 POINTS 1800-2000 = 1 POINT ABOVE 2000 = 0 POINTS	5 (1132)	1 (1653)	3 (1370)	5 (1080)	5 (1103)	3 (1446)	5 (1161)
TOTAL POINTS FOR THE DAY	31	14	29	31	29	27	33

TOTAL POINTS FOR THIS WEEK: ___194___
MAXIMUM POINTS FOR THIS WEEK: ___245___

Figure 3.6. Sample entry from the Daily Log measure of habit change and caloric intake.

From Brownell, K. D. *The partnership diet program.* New York: Rawson-Wade, 1980. Copyright © 1980 by Rawson-Wade Publishers. Reprinted by permission of the publisher.

Stimulus Control

Schachter (1971) and his colleagues (Schachter & Rodin, 1974) proposed that obese persons are extraordinarily responsive to food cues. These cues include time of day, the sight of food, and palatability. Schachter proposed that the obese person eats when exposed to food cues, independent of physiological hunger. The obvious implication for treatment is to teach the obese person to minimize exposure to food cues. Techniques designed for this purpose quickly became standard components of the behavior therapy program. Furthermore, the relative success of behavior therapy programs was cited as inferential evidence to support this "externality" hypothesis.

There is great debate about the externality theory (Rodin, 1978). Recent research is not entirely consistent, but it appears that obese and nonobese persons do not differ in their responsiveness to food cues (Rodin, 1980). Rodin (1980) has concluded that high sensitivity to food cues can be found in many persons in all weight categories. It is not known whether this sensitivity contributes to weight gain in the obese, or whether modification of this sensitivity can facilitate weight reduction. Behavior therapy studies are divided between those showing that stimulus-control techniques are useful (e.g., Beneke, Paulson, McReynolds, Lutz, & Kohrs, 1978) and those showing they are not (Loro, Fisher, & Levenkron, 1979). Until this issue is settled, stimulus-control procedures will continue as part of the behavioral program.

There are dozens of behaviors aimed at limiting exposure to food cues (Brownell, 1980). These can be classified into several broad categories: (1) keeping food out of sight; (2) limiting times and places that eating occurs as well as the activities associated with eating; (3) stopping "automatic" eating; (4) shopping prudently for food to keep problem foods out of the home; (5) avoiding dealing with food as much as possible.

Slowing the Rate of Eating

Decreasing eating rate may help the obese person control food intake, the theory being that less food will be eaten at the point when physiological satiety signals, "Halt eating." Again, it is not clear whether obese persons eat more rapidly than thin persons, whether rapid eating contributes to obesity, or whether slowing eating will aid in weight control. Despite these unanswered questions, behavioral programs encourage patients to slow the rate of eating by putting utensils down between bites, pausing in mid-meal, and in some cases, counting bites, chews, or swallows.

Reinforcement

Any behavior, including altered eating and exercise habits, must produce positive consequences (reinforcement) or it will not be sustained. Weight loss itself is usually not sufficient in this regard since most overweight persons lose weight, but inevitably return to their old habits.

The obese person is faced with a reinforcement imbalance. Figure 3.7 shows the positive and negative consequences facing a person who desires to eat but is attempting to lose weight. The rewards of eating are powerful and immediate; the food tastes good and it may relieve physical or emotional drives that make food attractive in the first place. In contrast, the negative consequences of eating are remote; these include guilt, poor health, and social distress. If the person exercises restraint and does not eat the food, the only reinforcers (satisfaction

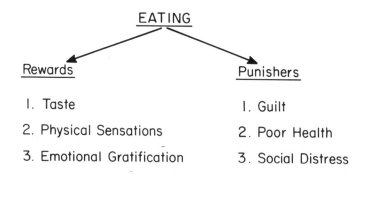

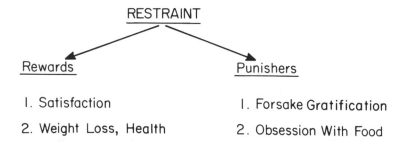

Figure 3.7. Rewards and punishers faced by the obese person deciding to eat or to restrain eating.

and the possible avoidance of health problems) are either weak or remote, and the punishers are powerful (forsaking taste, and being obsessed with the food). It is easy to see why the scale often tips in favor of eating.

There are several means by which desired behavior (restraint) can become more rewarding. Social rewards from a professional group leader or from peers in a treatment group are powerful motivators for appropriate eating and the resulting weight loss. Other social rewards may be available from the family or from other social groups, an issue discussed later. Self-determined rewards may also be useful. Some patients profit from structuring a formal reward system by which they administer themselves rewards contingent on behavior change or weight change. A simple example would be a person who "earns" points for each day at the desired calorie level, and then partakes in some enjoyable activity only when a specified number of points are earned. Finally, emotional self-rewards can be very powerful but may be difficult to teach. (This issue is discussed in the section on attitude restructuring in chapter 4.)

Nutrition

Many behavior therapy programs consider nutrition a secondary matter, because the focus should be on how the person eats, not what the person eats. I take a different view. The composition of the diet is an important factor in overall health, and obese persons are notorious for throwing nutritional wisdom to the winds when dieting. The first step in nutrition education is teaching the basic four food groups, or some alternative system of sensible eating. This is necessary for the patient to have a balanced diet but is not sufficient for weight loss to occur. For the obese person, nutrition education includes information on moderating salt intake, altering the balance of unsaturated to saturated fat, and insuring that adequate nutrients are consumed.

The behavior therapy program includes no specific diet, that is, no meal plans are provided. Prescribing a diet in which certain foods must be eaten and other foods are "illegal" sets the stage for the program to be abandoned when the inevitable transgressions occur. Patients are asked to limit their calories to 1200 per day for women and 1500 calories per day for men. These numbers are adjusted depending on each individual's energy balance, but the constitution of the diet, within the boundaries of good nutrition, is determined by the patient. This way, changes can be woven into a person's life-style—the only possible way for long-term change to occur.

Exercise/Physical Activity

There are four factors that make physical activity important in the treatment of obesity (Brownell & Stunkard, 1980): (1) energy expenditure; (2) appetite suppression; (3) remedy of the ill consequences of obesity; and (4) possible increases in basal metabolism. The first reason is most often proposed when advocating exercise for the obese, but the final three reasons may be much more important.

Energy expenditure. Increasing physical activity does increase energy expenditure, but not as much as many people think. For example, 1½ hours of brisk walking or running are necessary to expend the calories in a chocolate milkshake. Not only are many obese persons unwilling to devote the time to this type of exercise, many may not be capable of doing it. The caloric expense of exercise is likely to be beneficial when summing the cumulative effect of many small changes, not the short-term effect of major changes.

Appetite suppression. Weight loss in persons undertaking exercise programs is generally greater than would be expected from the energy expenditure caused by the increased activity. This suggests that activity may influence energy balance via its effect on food intake. In 1954, Mayer, Marshall, Vitale, Christensen, Mashayekhi, and Stare studied the effect on the food intake and body weight of rats forced to exercise. As shown in Figure 3.8, at most levels of exercise, food intake increased to compensate for increased energy output so that body weight remained stable. However, in the "sedentary" range of activity, food intake decreased as did body weight. Many subsequent studies confirmed this finding, and the effect seems to be more potent in obese than in lean animals (cf. Brownell & Stunkard, 1980). However, the effect varies with the sex of the animals (males do not compensate for increased expenditure, females do), the type of exercise, and the intensity of exercise.

Whether this appetite-suppression effect applies to humans is not known. Epstein, Masek, and Marshall (1978) found that food intake could be decreased in preschool children by changing recess from after lunch to before lunch. More research is needed in this important area, but an appetite-suppression effect of exercise is entirely possible.

Changing the consequences of obesity. Exercise may yield important benefits for the obese person even in the absence of weight loss. Exercise, in sufficient amounts, can favorably alter nearly every ill consequence of obesity. On the physiological side, exercise can lower blood pressure, change serum lipids, alter insulin sensitivity, and affect many other factors (Pollock, Wilmore, & Fox, 1978). Fox, Naughton,

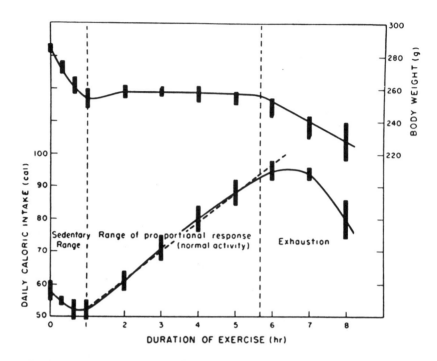

Figure 3.8.   Food intake and body weight as functions of duration of exercise in normal weight, female, adult rats.

From Mayer, J., Marshall, N. B., Vitale, J. J., Christensen, J. H., Mashayekhi, M. B., & Stare, F. J. Exercise, food intake, and body weight in normal rats and genetically obese adult mice. *American Journal of Physiology,* 1954, *177,* 544–548. Copyright © 1954 by the American Physiological Society. Reprinted by permission of the author and the publisher.

and Haskell (1971) have listed possible mechanisms by which exercise can influence the risk for coronary heart disease (Table 3.2). There are also potential psychological benefits from exercise. It may improve self-esteem, body image, and overall psychological functioning (Greist, Klein, Eischens, Faris, Gurman, & Morgan, 1979; Pollock et al., 1978).

Basal metabolism.   Basal metabolism accounts for the majority of the body's total energy expenditure (Astrand & Rodahl, 1977; Bray, 1976). Slight shifts in basal metabolism can have a large influence on body weight. Unfortunately for the dieter, basal metabolism decreases with the onset of caloric deprivation (Bray, 1976; Wooley, Wooley, & Dyrenforth, 1979). This decrease in basal metabolism is detectable within 48 hours of caloric restriction and can reach 20 percent within

Table 3.2 Mechanisms by which Physical Activity May Reduce the Occurrence and Severity of Coronary Heart Disease

Increase	Decrease
Coronary collateral vascularization	Serum lipid levels
Vessel size	Cholesterol
Myocardial efficiency	Triglycerides
Efficiency of peripheral blood	Glucose intolerance
distribution and return	Obesity-adiposity
Electron transport capacity	Platelet stickiness
Fibrinolytic capacity	Arterial blood pressure
Red blood cell mass and blood volume	Heart rate
Thyroid function	Vulnerability to dysrhythmias
Growth hormone production	Neurohormonal overreaction
Tolerance to stress	"Strain" associated with "psychic
Prudent living habits	stress"
"Joie de vivre"	

From Fox, S. M., III, Naughton, J. P., & Haskell, W. L. Physical activity and the prevention of coronary heart disease. *Annals of Clinical Research,* 1971, *3,* 404–432. Copyright © 1971 by the Finnish Medical Society Dvodecim. Reprinted by permission of the author and the Editor-in-Chief.

14 days. Figure 3.9 shows that this decrease proceeds even faster than weight loss. Furthermore, successive episodes of dieting are accompanied by more rapid decreases in basal metabolism and by slower recovery to baseline levels when caloric deprivation is terminated (Bray, 1976; Brownell & Stunkard, 1980; Wooley et al., 1979). The consequence is clear; weight reduction creates adaptive changes that retard further weight reduction. There is some evidence that exercise can help offset this decrease (Mayer, 1968; Scheuer & Tipton, 1977), but this fact has not been clearly documented.

The Results of Behavior Therapy

A wealth of information is available on behavior therapy for obesity. The highlights of this information will be presented here, because comprehensive reviews are available elsewhere (Foreyt, 1977; Mahoney, 1978; Stunkard, 1975; Stunkard & Mahoney, 1976; Stunkard & Penick, 1979; Wilson, 1980; Wilson & Brownell, 1980).

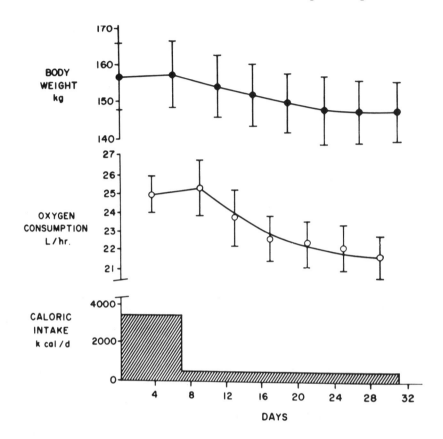

Figure 3.9.   Effect of caloric restriction on oxygen consumption of six obese patients. After one week on a diet of 3500 kcal/day, caloric intake was reduced to 450 kcal/day. Body weight declined, but the drop in oxygen intake was proportionally faster, representing a fall of 15 percent by the end of two weeks.

From Bray, G. A. Effect of caloric restriction on energy expenditure in obese patients. *Lancet*, 1969, *2*, 397–398. Copyright © 1969 *The Lancet*. Reprinted by permission of the author and the publisher.

Attrition, Psychological Factors, and Methodology Issues

Behavior therapy can claim several major accomplishments aside from the issue of weight loss. First, attrition in behavior-therapy programs averages approximately 12 percent (Wilson & Brownell, 1980). This is impressive compared to the 50 to 80 percent attrition reported for other forms of treatment (Stunkard & Brownell, 1979). Attrition may be the most important adherence issue facing obesity researchers today, so the low attrition rates from behavioral programs are noteworthy. Parenthetically, estimates of weight losses from behavior-therapy programs are probably biased in a conservative direction, because unsuccessful patients who drop out of other programs are typically retained in behavioral programs. Adherence issues will be discussed in greater detail in Chapter 4.

The second accomplishment of behavior therapy has been a dramatic reduction in the untoward emotional consequences of dieting. As mentioned earlier, dieting is associated with a number of emotional symptoms. Behavioral programs have not reported these emotional symptoms. In fact, in studies where careful assessment of emotional response has been undertaken, behavior therapy appears to produce *improvement* in psychological functioning (Brownell & Stunkard, 1981; Craighead et al., 1980; Taylor, Ferguson, & Reading, 1978).

Behavior therapy researchers have brought great experimental rigor to the study of treatments for obesity. Prior to the proliferation of behavior therapy studies, uncontrolled case reports were the rule. Now, well-controlled investigations are being conducted with large subject populations, low attrition, and long-term follow-up.

Short-term Weight Loss

In 1978 Jeffery, Wing, and Stunkard published a review of 21 studies of behavior therapy for obesity. The mean weight loss in programs ranging from eight to 12 weeks in duration was 11.5 pounds. These same authors presented data on the first 125 patients who entered the Stanford Eating Disorders Clinic; the average loss was 11.04 pounds. Brownell, Heckerman, and Westlake (1979) studied 100 obese patients in their clinic at Brown University and reported an average weight loss of 11.01 pounds. In 1979 Stunkard and Penick reviewed ten behavior therapy studies with follow-ups of one year or longer. The mean weight loss after a treatment period averaging 11 weeks was 11.7 pounds. Wilson and Brownell (1980) conducted an even more recent review of the 17 existing long-term studies and found average weight losses of 10.4 pounds during programs averaging 12.8 weeks. These results are remarkably consistent, despite variations across programs in demographic factors for the patients, training of the therapists, amount of treatment fees, and specifics of the treatment program.

How meaningful is an average weight loss of 11 pounds in an

11-week treatment program? First, there is enormous variability around this mean loss, that is, some patients lose much more and some lose much less (Wilson & Brownell, 1980). Second, the goal of behavior therapy is a weight loss of one to two pounds per week, so the average loss of 11 pounds in 11 weeks is not surprising. Third, compared to the paltry losses reported for other treatments, the statistical effect of behavior therapy is robust (Jeffery et al., 1978). However, an 11-pound loss for the average patient who weighs 50 to 70 pounds too much is not impressive. The final judgment depends on results over the long term. Do patients maintain their losses, or, even more important, do they continue losing weight?

Long-term Weight Loss

In the review of long-term studies by Stunkard and Penick (1979), the average posttreatment loss of 11.7 pounds had decreased only slightly (to 10.9 pounds) after a one-year follow-up. In a follow-up of their own patients, reported on earlier by Penick, Filion, Fox, and Stunkard (1971), the posttreatment weight loss of 22.2 pounds actually increased (to 27.7 pounds) at a one-year follow-up. However, Stunkard and Penick conclude that losses in behavior-therapy programs are only "modestly maintained," perhaps because the five-year follow-up of their patients revealed an average loss of 11.7 pounds.

Wilson and Brownell (1980), in their review of 17 controlled studies with a one-year follow-up, found almost no change in the mean weight loss from posttreatment (10.4 pounds) to follow-up (10.2 pounds). There are reports of larger weight losses and somewhat better maintenance in uncontrolled studies (Wilson & Brownell, 1980), but these need to be confirmed by controlled research.

It can be concluded that behavior therapy produces average losses of one pound per week during programs that average 11 weeks in duration. It appears that the losses increase if patients are treated for more than 11 weeks, but programs have not yet gone beyond 25 weeks (Brownell & Stunkard, 1981; Craighead et al. 1980; Jeffery et al., 1978). The losses produced in treatment are very well maintained on the average, but the average patient does not continue to lose weight during follow-up. Compared with other treatments, behavior therapy is very effective, but considering the amount of weight most patients need to lose, we have much to learn about developing a successful treatment. This fact has prompted some researchers to move beyond the standard behavioral program in search of more innovative and effective approaches.

New Developments in Behavioral Treatments

This section will cover two of the most promising new developments in behavior therapy for obesity: combining pharmacotherapy with behavior therapy and couples treatment. There are other encouraging approaches, such as combining behavior therapy with dietary interventions (Bistrian, 1978), giving more emphasis to exercise (Dahlkoetter, Callahan, & Linton, 1979), and using multifaceted treatment programs in residential settings (Miller & Simms, 1981). These advances have been reviewed elsewhere (Brownell & Venditti, in press; Stunkard, 1980; Wilson & Brownell, 1980).

Combining Behavior Therapy with Pharmacotherapy

Pharmacotherapy for obesity began its popularity more than 40 years ago. In recent times this approach has fallen into disrepute because of short-lived weight losses and the abuse potential of many drugs, particularly the amphetamines. There are, however, several drugs that are relatively safe and have the potential for enhancing weight loss. Combining the pharmacological approach with behavior therapy might be a useful endeavor if the habit change produced by behavior therapy could sustain the weight lost via drugs.

Craighead and colleagues (1980) tested behavior therapy in conjunction with fenfluramine, a sympathomimetic amine with sedative properties. Subjects were assigned to four treatment conditions: (1) routine doctor's office treatment with fenfluramine; (2) behavior therapy in groups; (3) fenfluramine with Rogerian nondirective therapy in groups; and (4) fenfluramine combined with group behavior therapy. After 25 weekly sessions, the mean weight losses for the four conditions were 14.1, 24, 30, and 31.9 pounds, respectively (Figure 3.10: weight given in kilograms). These data suggest that pharmacotherapy can lead to substantial weight loss if administered in the context of group therapy. Adding behavior therapy to pharmacotherapy improved the weight loss somewhat, and the medication (with or without behavior therapy) was more effective than behavior therapy alone.

The follow-up results in this study showed a clear reversal in the long-term effectiveness of pharmacotherapy and behavior therapy (Figure 3.10). At a one-year follow-up, the doctor's office subjects had received other treatment. The mean weight losses for the remaining conditions were 20 pounds for group behavior therapy, 14.1 pounds for drug plus nondirective group treatment, and 10.1 pounds for the

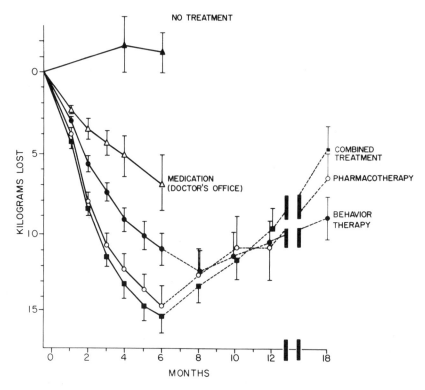

Figure 3.10. Mean weight change in kilograms for the experimental groups receiving fenfluramine, behavior therapy, or their combination.

From Craighead, L. W., Stunkard, A. J., & O'Brien, R. Behavior therapy and pharmacotherapy of obesity. *Lancet,* 1980, *2,* 1045–1047. Copyright © 1981 *The Lancet.* Reprinted by permission of the author and the publisher.

combination of behavior therapy and pharmacotherapy. Subjects receiving the behavior therapy alone regained little weight, whereas subjects receiving the drug rebounded rapidly. Surprisingly, subjects who received both treatments rebounded as rapidly as subjects who received only the drug. Craighead and co-workers concluded that the drug compromised the effects of behavior therapy.

Combining Couples Training with Pharmacotherapy

Craighead and associates (1980) showed that pharmacotherapy could produce large and rapid weight losses but that these losses were poorly maintained. Furthermore, behavior therapy alone was not effective in preventing the relapse that occurred after the drug was discontinued. Brownell and co-workers (1978) found that a couples training program could produce impressive initial losses. These losses were not only well-maintained, but subjects actually lost additional weight during follow-up. Combining these two approaches was the next logical step, in hopes of encouraging large losses via the drug and then sustaining the losses by working with the social environment.

Brownell and Stunkard (1981) used a 3 × 2 experimental design (shown below) to test couples training and pharmacotherapy, alone and in combination. A total of 124 obese patients were randomly assigned to one of six conditions. The spouse conditions were identical to those used in the study of Brownell and colleagues (1978), and, in addition, subjects were randomly assigned to receive fenfluramine or no drug. A total of 124 subjects were treated with 16 weekly sessions and then with booster sessions every other month for the year following treatment.

Design for Brownell & Stunkard (1981) Study

	Drug	*No Drug*
Couples Training		
Cooperative Spouse,		
Subject Alone		
Uncooperative Spouse		

Results for subjects receiving fenfluramine and those not receiving medication replicate the findings of Craighead and associates (1980). Figure 3.11 shows that drug subjects lost significantly more weight during treatment (24 pounds) than did no-drug subjects (17 pounds). (Figure 3.11 gives weight in kilograms.) At follow-up, however, subjects who received fenfluramine regained weight much more rapidly than did no-drug subjects, so that one year after treatment, there were no statistical differences between the two conditions.

The results from the couples conditions were most surprising. Figure 3.12 shows that the three couples conditions did not differ significantly after treatment or follow-up. The three spouse conditions showed equivalent weight losses during initial treatment, and there were no differences in the maintenance of loss among the conditions. The couples training was not more effective than the two control conditions in sustaining the weight loss via pharmacotherapy, and the interactions between drug and spouse conditions were not significant.

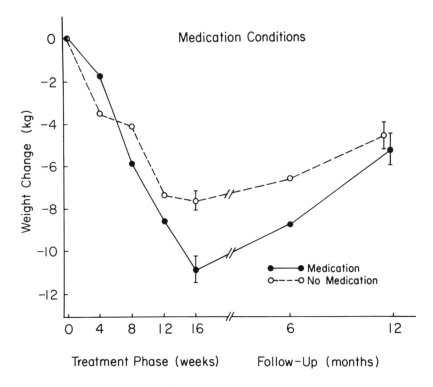

Figure 3.11. Mean weight change in kilograms for medication (fenfluramine) and no-medication groups. Data are collapsed across the three couples conditions.

The fact that the couples-training condition did not help maintain the drug-produced loss is not surprising, considering that the couples-training subjects did no better than subjects in the two control conditions. It *is* surprising that the couples-training program differed so markedly from the program reported by Brownell and colleagues (1978). Brownell and Stunkard (1981) attribute this to differences in the subject populations. These authors propose more research on the interactions among dieters and their spouses to learn more about attitudes, shared eating patterns, mutual coping skills, and so forth.

From this series of three studies we can conclude that pharmacotherapy is a powerful method of promoting initial weight loss. The problem of relapse has not been solved, and two promising means of accomplishing long-term maintenance (behavior therapy and couples training) have not been effective. Couples training has also been very

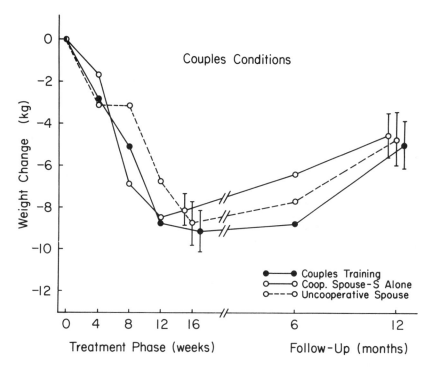

Figure 3.12.   Mean weight change in kilograms for the three couples conditions
of spouse intervention. Data are collapsed across drug and no-
drug conditions.

effective in some studies, but not in others. Undoubtedly, further
understanding of marital relations and how to structure couples techniques will produce more consistent results with this approach.

Conclusion

Obesity is a problem that combines extreme seriousness, alarming
prevalence, and striking resistance to treatment. Behavior therapy, the
only therapy to be evaluated extensively, is more effective than the
alternative treatments to which it has been compared. Weight losses
from behavior therapy average 11 pounds in programs that average 11
weeks in duration. The long-term results are more favorable than
previously believed; average losses after 12 months of follow-up tend

to be approximately 10 to 11 pounds. This makes behavior therapy the most effective nonsurgical procedure for the treatment of obesity, and so it should be considered the treatment of choice for mild to moderate obesity. There is much to be learned, however, considering that the average patient may have at least 50 pounds to lose. Two promising developments in treatment (couples training and pharmacotherapy) show great potential, but more research is needed before this potential can be realized.

References

Abraham, S., & Nordsieck, M. Relationship of excess weight in children and adults. *Public Health Reports,* 1960, *75,* 263–273.

Ashby, W. A., & Wilson, G. T. Behavior therapy for obesity: Booster sessions and long-term maintenance of weight loss. *Behavior Research and Therapy,* 1977, *15,* 451–464.

Astrand, P. O., & Rodahl, K. *Textbook of work physiology.* New York: McGraw-Hill, 1977.

Bandura, A. *Principles of behavior modification.* New York: Holt, Rinehart, & Winston, 1969.

Beaumont, W. *Experiments and observations on the gastric juice and the physiology of digestion.* New York: Dover Publications, 1959.

Beneke, W. M., Paulson, B., McReynolds, W. T., Lutz, R. N., & Kohrs, M. B. Long-term results of two behavior modification weight loss programs using nutritionists as therapists. *Behavior Therapy,* 1978, *9,* 501–507.

Bistrian, B. R. Clinical use of a protein-sparing modified fast. *Journal of the American Medical Association,* 1978, *21,* 2299–2302.

Bray, G. A. *The obese patient.* Philadelphia: Saunders, 1976.

Bray, G. A. (Ed.). *Obesity in America.* U.S. Department of Health, Education, and Welfare. National Institutes of Health, NIH Publication No. 79–359, 1979.

Brownell, K. D. *Behavior therapy for weight control: A treatment manual.* Unpublished manuscript, University of Pennsylvania, 1979.

Brownell, K. D. *The partnership diet program.* New York: Rawson-Wade, 1980.

Brownell, K. D., Heckerman, C. L., & Westlake, R. J. The behavioral control of obesity. A descriptive analysis of a large-scale program. *Journal of Clinical Psychology,* 1979, *35,* 864–869.

Brownell, K. D., Heckerman, C. L., Westlake, R. J., Hayes, S. C., & Monti, P. M. The effect of couples training and partner cooperativeness in the behavioral treatment of obesity. *Behavior Research and Therapy,* 1978, *16,* 323–333.

Brownell, K. D., & Stunkard, A. J. Behavioral treatment of obesity in children. *American Journal of Diseases of Children,* 1978, *132,* 403–412.

Brownell, K. D., & Stunkard, A. J. Exercise in the development and control of obesity. In A. J. Stunkard (Ed.), *Obesity*. Philadelphia: Saunders, 1980.

Brownell, K. D., & Stunkard, A. J. Couples training, pharmacotherapy, and behavior therapy in the treatment of obesity. *Archives of General Psychiatry*, 1981, *38*, 1224–1229.

Brownell, K. D., & Venditti, E. M. The etiology and treatment of obesity. In W. E. Fann, I. Karacan, A. D. Pokorny, & R. L. Williams (Eds.), *Phenomenology and the treatment of psychophysiological disorders*. New York: Spectrum, in press.

Chiang, B. N., Perlman, L. V., & Epstein, F. H. Overweight and hypertension: A review. *Circulation*, 1969, *39*, 403–421.

Craighead, L. W., Stunkard, A. J., & O'Brien, R. Behavior therapy and pharmacotherapy of obesity. *Lancet*, 1980, *2*, 1045–1047.

Dahlkoetter, J., Callahan, E. J., & Linton, J. Obesity and the unbalanced energy equation: Exercise vs. eating habit change. *Journal of Consulting and Clinical Psychology*, 1979, *47*, 898–905.

Drash, A. Relationship between diabetes mellitus and obesity in the child. *Metabolism*, 1973, *22*, 337–344.

Dwyer, J., & Mayer, J. The dismal condition: Problems faced by obese adolescent girls in American society. In G. Bray (Ed.), *Obesity in perspective*. Bethesda, Md.: DHEW Publication No. (NIH) 75–708, 1975.

Epstein, L. H., Masek, B., & Marshall, W. Pre-lunch exercise and lunchtime caloric intake. *Behavior Therapist*, 1978, *1*, 15.

Eysenck, H. J. Learning theory and behavior therapy. *Journal of Mental Science*, 1959, *105*, 61–75.

Ferguson, J. M. *Learning to eat: Behavior modification for weight control*. Palo Alto, Calif.: Bull, 1975.

Foreyt, J. P. (Ed.), *Behavioral treatments of obesity*. New York: Pergamon, 1977.

Fox, S. M., III, Naughton, J. P., & Haskell, W. L. Physical activity in the prevention of coronary heart disease. *Annals of Clinical Research*, 1971, *3*, 404–432.

Garn, S. M., & Clark, D. C. Trends in fatness and the origins of obesity. *Pediatrics*, 1976, *57*, 443–456.

Gordon, T., Castelli, W. P., Hjortland, M. C., Kannel, W. B., & Dawber, T. R. Diabetes, blood lipids and the role of obesity in coronary heart disease risk for women. *Annals of Internal Medicine*, 1977, *87*, 393–397.

Gordon, T., & Kannel, W. B. The effects of overweight on cardiovascular disease. *Geriatrics*, 1973, *28*, 80–88.

Greist, J. H., Klein, M. H., Eischens, R. R., Faris, J., Gurman, A. S., & Morgan, W. P. Running as treatment for depression. *Comprehensive Psychiatry*, 1979, *20*, 41–54.

Jeffery, R. W., Wing, R. R., & Stunkard, A. J. Behavioral treatment of obesity: The state of the art in 1976. *Behavior Therapy*, 1978, *9*, 189–199.

Jeffrey, D. B., & Katz, R. C. *Take it off and keep it off: A behavioral program for weight loss and healthy living*. Englewood Cliffs, N.J.: Prentice-Hall, 1977.

Jordan, H. A., Levitz, L. S., & Kimbrell, G. M. *Eating is okay: A radical approach to weight loss, the behavioral control diet.* New York: Rawson-Wade, 1977.

Kannel, W. B., & Gordon, T. Physiological and medical concomitants of obesity: The Framingham Study. In G. A. Bray (Ed.), *Obesity in America.* Washington, D.C.: U.S. Department of Health, Education and Welfare, NIH Publication No. 79–359, 1979.

Kannel, W. B., Gordon, T., & Castelli, W. P. Obesity, lipids and glucose intolerance: The Framingham Study. *American Journal of Clinical Nutrition,* 1979, *32,* 1238–1245.

Kingsley, R. G., & Wilson, G. T. Behavior therapy for obesity: A comparative investigation of long-term efficacy. *Journal of Consulting and Clinical Psychology,* 1977, *45,* 288–298.

Loro, A. D., Jr., Fisher, E. B., Jr., & Levenkron, J. C. Comparison of established and innovative weight-reduction treatment procedures. *Journal of Applied Behavior Analysis,* 1979, *12,* 141–155.

Maddox, G. L., Back, K. W., & Liederman, V. R. Overweight as social deviance and disability. *Journal of Health and Social Behavior,* 1968, *9,* 287–298.

Mahoney, M. J. Behavior modification in the treatment of obesity. *Psychiatric Clinics of North America,* 1978, *1,* 651–660.

Mahoney, M. J., & Mahoney, K. *Permanent weight control: A total solution to the dieter's dilemma,* New York: Norton, 1976.

Mann, G. V. The influence of obesity on health. *New England Journal of Medicine,* 1974, *291,* 178–185, 226–232.

Mayer, J. *Overweight: Causes, cost, and control.* Englewood Cliffs, N.J.: Prentice-Hall, 1968.

Mayer, J., Marshall, N. B., Vitale, J. J., Christensen, J. H., Mashayekhi, M. B., & Stare, F. J. Exercise, food intake, and body weight in normal rats and genetically obese adult mice. *American Journal of Physiology,* 1954, *177,* 544–548.

Miller, P. M., & Simms, K. L. Evaluation and component analysis of a comprehensive weight control program. *International Journal of Obesity,* 1981, *5,* 57–66.

Penick, S. B., Filion, R., Fox, S., & Stunkard, A. J. Behavior modification in the treatment of obesity. *Psychosomatic Medicine,* 1971, *33,* 49–55.

Pollock, M. L., Wilmore, J. H., & Fox, S. M., III. *Health and fitness through physical activity.* New York: Wiley, 1978.

Richardson, S. A., Hastorf, A. J., Goodman, N., Dornbush, S. S. Cultural uniformity in reaction to physical disabilities. *American Sociological Review,* 1961, *26,* 241–247.

Rodin, J. Environmental factors in obesity. *Psychiatric Clinics of North America,* 1978, *1,* 581–592.

Rodin, J. The externality theory today. In A. J. Stunkard (Ed.), *Obesity.* Philadelphia: Saunders, 1980.

Schachter, S. Some extraordinary facts about obese humans and rats. *American Psychologist,* 1971, *26,* 129–144.

Schachter, S., & Rodin, J. *Obese humans and rats.* Washington, D.C.: Erlbaum/ Halsted, 1974.

Scheuer, J., & Tipton, C. M. Cardiovascular adaptations to physical training. *Annual Review of Physiology,* 1977, *39,* 221–251.

Silverstone, J. P., & Lascelles, B. D. Dieting and depression. *British Journal of Psychiatry,* 1966, *112,* 513–519.

Skinner, B. F. *Science and human behavior.* New York: Macmillan, 1953.

Staffieri, J. R. A study of social stereotype of body image in children. *Journal of Personality and Social Psychology,* 1967, *7,* 101–104.

Stuart, R. B. Behavioral control of overeating. *Behavior Research and Therapy,* 1967, *5,* 357–365.

Stuart, R. B. *Act thin, stay thin.* New York: Norton, 1978.

Stuart, R. B., & Davis, B. *Slim chance in a fat world: Behavioral control of obesity.* Champaign, Ill.: Research Press, 1972.

Stunkard, A. J. The dieting depression: Incidence and clinical characteristics of untoward responses to weight reduction regimens. *American Journal of Medicine,* 1957, *23,* 77–86.

Stunkard, A. J. From explanation to action in psychosomatic medicine: The case of obesity. *Psychosomatic Medicine,* 1975, *37,* 195–236.

Stunkard, A. J. *The pain of obesity.* Palo Alto, Calif.: Bull, 1976.

Stunkard, A. J. (Ed.). *Obesity.* Philadelphia: Saunders, 1980.

Stunkard, A. J., & Brownell, K. D. Behavior therapy and self-help programs for obesity. In J. F. Munro (Ed.), *The treatment of obesity.* London: MTP Press, 1979.

Stunkard, A. J., & Burt, V. Obesity and the body image. II. Age at onset of disturbances in the body image. *American Journal of Psychiatry,* 1967, *123,* 1443–1447.

Stunkard, A. J., & Mahoney, M. J. Behavioral treatment of eating disorders. In H. Leitenberg (Ed.), *The handbook of behavior modification.* Englewood Cliffs, N.J.: Prentice-Hall, 1976.

Stunkard, A. J., & Mendelson, M. Obesity and body image: I. Characteristics of disturbances in the body image of some obese persons. *American Journal of Psychiatry,* 1967, *123,* 1296–1300.

Stunkard, A. J., & Penick, S. B. Behavior modification in the treatment of obesity: The problem of maintaining weight loss. *Archives of General Psychiatry,* 1979, *36,* 801–806.

Stunkard, A. J., & Rush, A. J. Dieting and depression reexamined: A critical review of reports of untoward responses during weight reduction for obesity. *Annals of Internal Medicine,* 1974, *81,* 526–533.

Taylor, C. B., Ferguson, J. M., & Reading, J. C. Gradual weight loss and depression. *Behavior Therapy,* 1978, *9,* 622–625.

United States Senate Select Subcommittee on Nutrition and Human Needs. Proceedings from hearings. U.S. Government Printing Office, 1977.

Van Itallie, T. B. Obesity: Adverse effects on health and longevity. *American Journal of Clinical Nutrition,* 1979, *32,* 2723–2733.

Wilson, G. T. Behavior therapy for obesity. In A. J. Stunkard (Ed.), *Obesity.* Philadelphia: Saunders, 1980.

Wilson, G. T., & Brownell, K. D. Behavior therapy for obesity: Including family members in the treatment process. *Behavior Therapy,* 1978, *9,* 943–945.

Wilson, G. T., & Brownell, K. D. Behavior therapy for obesity: An evaluation of treatment outcome. *Advances in Behavior Research and Therapy,* 1980, *3,* 49–86.

Wilson, G. T., & O'Leary, K. D. *Principles of behavior therapy.* Englewood Cliffs, N.J.: Prentice-Hall, 1980.

Wolpe, J. *Psychotherapy by reciprocal inhibition.* Stanford, Calif.: Stanford University Press, 1958.

Wooley, S. C., Wooley, O. W., & Dyrenforth, S. R. Theoretical, practical, and social issues in behavioral treatments of obesity. *Journal of Applied Behavior Analysis,* 1979, *12,* 3–26.

4

Obesity: Treatment Effectiveness and Adherence to Behavioral Programs

Kelly D. Brownell

Thirty percent of all American men and 40 percent of all women between the ages of 40 and 49 are considered obese by the criterion of being at least 20 percent above ideal weight (Metropolitan Life Insurance Company, 1960). The prevalence is even higher among persons in lower socioeconomic groups (Goldblatt, Moore, & Stunkard, 1965), with advancing age (Build and Blood Pressure Study, 1959), and in a variety of ethnic groups (Stunkard, 1975). Since 1900 the prevalence of obesity has doubled (Waxler & Leef, 1969); and the Build and Blood Pressure Study (1959) and the Health and Nutrition Survey (1976) showed continuing weight gains in Americans in the past 27 years. The U.S. Department of Health, Education and Welfare (1966) has labeled obesity the number one dietary problem.

For many years, few questioned that obesity was a serious disorder. Recently, however, skeptics have become more fearful, particularly in public circles and in the scientific community. One lay group, the National Association to Aid Fat Americans, maintains that some persons may lead more fulfilling lives if they are overweight and that society should be educated to cease discriminating against fat people

Portions reprinted with permission of the author from *National Institute on Drug Abuse Research Monograph*, No. 25, DHEW No. ADM 79–839, U.S. Government Printing Office, Washington, D.C., June 1979.

society should be educated to cease discriminating against fat people rather than advocating dieting at any cost. This movement has gained momentum, despite mounting evidence that obesity carries a high risk of physical and psychological problems.

Obesity is strongly associated with several established precursors to coronary heart disease, including hypertension, increased low-density lipoproteins and decreased high-density lipoprotein cholesterol, hypertriglyceridemia, increased insulin production, and impaired glucose tolerance (Kannel & Gordon, 1979). There is some dispute as to whether obesity is a risk factor independent of its association with other risk factors (Mann, 1974), yet it seems certain that obesity is medically undesirable. Data from the Framingham Study indicate that if everyone were at optimal weight, there would be 25 percent less coronary heart disease and 35 percent fewer episodes of congestive heart failure and cerebrovascular accidents (Gordon & Kannel, 1976). Kannel & Gordon (1979) have gone even further, to claim that " . . . correction of overweight is probably the most important hygienic measure (aside from avoidance of cigarettes) available for the control of cardiovascular disease" (p. 140).

There have been innumerable attempts to help overweight persons lose weight. Some are scientifically sound; most are not. A glance into almost any popular magazine reveals diets that promise miraculous weight loss, happiness, and sexiness. Diets, pills, devices, and spiritual plans—many of which defy reason—are commercially successful. This may be testimony to how desperate many obese persons are to reduce and to how little confidence they have in scientists to help them achieve this goal. Are they right?

I will give a brief history of the treatment of obesity, concentrating on recent evidence of effectiveness of behavioral approaches. A new concept for the treatment of obesity based on adherence problems will be offered.

How Effective Is Treatment?

There are hundreds of "guaranteed" cures for obesity. One need look no farther than the shelves of supermarkets or bookstores to find countless remedies, each of which makes bold claims about the miracles awaiting the obese person. These approaches range from pills that will "melt fat" to sweat suits that attach with a hose to a vacuum cleaner.

These miracle cures are commercially successful—witness their ubiquity and their staying power in the marketplace. One wonders why the obese purchase devices that strain the imagination, particularly when they are the first to admit that such devices are worthless. Stunkard & Brownell (1979) note:

> Why is there such a booming market for weight reduction methods? The answer seems clear: millions are plagued by excess weight. Many attempt to reduce by methods that are largely ineffective. Confronted by failure, they move on to another approach and then another, creating a lucrative market for those who promise what cannot be delivered. The fact that so many overweight people are attracted to such questionable measures is testimony to how desperately they want to lose weight and how difficult it is for them to do so. Millions more have given up even trying [p. 199].

Can we infer that professional treatments are not effective, and that obese persons resort to exploitative schemes as a result of disenchantment with other approaches? If "cure" from obesity is defined as reduction to ideal weight and maintenance of that weight for five years, a person is more likely to recover from almost any form of cancer than from obesity (Van Itallie, 1977).

Almost 25 years ago, Stunkard (1958) issued a most pessimistic verdict: "Most obese persons will not enter treatment for obesity. Of those who enter treatment, most will not lose weight and of those who do lose weight, most will regain it" (p. 86). From 20 to 80 percent of obese persons were found to drop out of traditional medical treatment programs, and of the few persons left, fewer than 25 percent lost as much as 20 lbs. (9.1 kg); only 5 percent lost as much as 40 lbs. (18.2 kg) (Stunkard & McLaren-Hume, 1959). To make matters worse, emotional symptoms have been documented in at least 50 percent of persons treated for obesity by either outpatient dieting or inpatient fasting (Stunkard & Rush, 1974).

In 1967 Stuart brought new hope to this discouraging area. In a study entitled "The Behavioral Control of Overeating," Stuart reported the results of a yearlong, multifaceted behavioral treatment program for eight subjects. Even though Stuart's results were from uncontrolled case studies, the weight losses were impressive enough to spur dozens of later studies: 30 percent of Stuart's subjects lost more than 40 lbs. (18.2 kg) and 60 percent lost more than 30 lbs. (13.6 kg).

Until recently, Stuart's treatment procedures—known as the behavioral package—have remained unchallenged and have been used in nearly every study on the behavioral treatment of obesity. In the years since Stuart's work, there have been major advances in our understanding of treatment techniques. The first logical step was to determine whether Stuart's subjects would have improved without treatment.

Harris (1969) addressed this question by assigning subjects to behavioral groups or to a no-treatment control group. Subjects given behavioral treatment lost more weight than control subjects and even continued losing weight after treatment ended. Wollersheim (1970) then compared behavior therapy to placebo conditions and found that behavior therapy was more effective. Both Harris and Wollersheim significantly improved treatment methods, and it appeared that behavior therapy was better than other available approaches. The effect of experimenter bias in these studies could not be ruled out; it is possible that enthusiastic doctoral students in behavioral programs could have influenced the outcome of their studies.

A study by Penick, Filion, Fox, and Stunkard (1971) attempted to control for experimenter bias by biasing the outcome against the behavioral approach. In this study, behavioral groups were conducted by inexperienced therapists and traditional treatment groups were conducted by therapists with much experience. The behavioral groups still did better. This study strengthened the belief that behavior therapy was the most effective approach for obesity and suggested that this type of therapy could be carried out by persons with little training or experience.

The possibility that the content of behavioral programs was more important than the quality of the therapist prompted several researchers to investigate therapy without a therapist. Hagen (1974) replicated Wollersheim's (1970) treatment program under two conditions: group treatment led by a trained clinician, and a bibliotherapy condition in which subjects received a written manual via mail, with little therapist contact. Both treatments were equally effective and were superior to a no-treatment control condition. Similar studies by Ferstl, Jokusch, & Brengelman 1975) in Germany and by Hanson, Borden, Hall, and Hall (1976) in the United States also showed that bibliotherapy was as effective as group therapy.

In contrast to these three studies, Brownell, Heckerman, and Westlake (1978a) found that bibliotherapy was less effective than group therapy, although weight losses in both groups were not maintained. This suggested that the amount of contact may be an important variable. Fernan (1973) answered this question by comparing minimal contact to no contact. The results showed that even minimal contact was more useful than no contact. It can tentatively be concluded, therefore, that any therapist contact is better than no contact, but that after this minimal amount, additional therapist time may be of little use.

The next logical step was to concentrate on technique refinement. The behavioral package was thought to be effective, so research could focus on determining the active components of the multifaceted package or on enhancing the efficacy of any single component. Several studies, for example, evaluated the influence of self-monitoring (Green, 1978; Romanczyk, 1974; Romanczyck, Tracey, Wilson, & Thorpe, 1973). Others investigated self-reinforcement (Mahoney, 1974), goal setting (Bandura & Simon, 1977), covert sensitization (Diament & Wilson, 1975; Foreyt & Hagen, 1973; Foreyt & Kennedy, 1971), exercise (Harris & Hallbauer, 1973; Stalonas, Johnson, & Christ, 1978), and so forth. The result has been a great improvement in treatment-outcome research but little improvement in treatment efficacy. Indeed, no studies have even approached Stuart's (1967) impressive results. How effective, then, is behavior therapy for obesity?

Jeffery, Wing, and Stunkard (1978) reviewed the results from 21 studies of behavioral treatment procedures and found an average weight loss of 11.5 lbs. (5.2 kg). The same authors reported the results for 125 patients from the Stanford Eating Disorders Clinic; average weight loss was 11.04 lbs. (5 kg). Brownell, Heckerman, and Westlake (1976) studied 98 subjects in a behavioral weight-loss program and found an average weight loss of 11.01 lbs. (5 kg).

The consistency of weight losses is striking considering that the studies differed widely in length of treatment, therapist training, patient characteristics, treatment fees, and a variety of program variables. We can predict with great certainty how much weight the average subject will lose in a behavioral treatment program; the ability of subjects to maintain their weight losses is another question.

The typical treatment outcome study provides follow-up data for six to eight weeks. Even for such short follow-up periods, maintenance of weight losses has been conspicuously lacking. In a recent review of long-term studies, Stunkard and Penick (1979) found that maintenance of weight loss has been exceedingly rare. There have been surprisingly few attempts to study the maintenance problem. The exception is a series of studies on booster sessions by Wilson and colleagues (Ashby & Wilson, 1977; Kingsley & Wilson, 1977; Wilson & Brownell, 1978). Since treatment-produced weight losses usually dissipate when sessions end, and since Stuart had achieved good results from continued contact with his patients over a one-year period, booster sessions after treatment held the promise of enhancing maintenance. Unfortunately, the studies found that booster sessions were not effective in maintaining weight loss for subjects receiving group behavioral treatment, although booster sessions did seem to be effective for subjects in individual treatment.

Behavioral treatments are more effective at producing initial weight loss than are other treatments to which they have been compared, although the clinical significance of the weight losses can be questioned. The maintenance of weight loss on a long-term basis is an elusive goal, and few treatment strategies have been effective for approaching it. It would appear, therefore, that maintenance of treatment-produced behavior changes is presently an area of great importance. However, increasing initial weight loss is also important if we wish to aid any but the most modestly obese.

Progress in approaching obesity and other health behavior changes requires a different conceptual viewpoint; this new conceptual scheme may prompt the use of behavioral procedures for a critical problem: program adherence.

Obesity as an Adherence Problem

Most professionals approach weight loss by instructing the obese in *what* to eat. Health care professionals, in cases where they offer anything more than exhortation, typically give the obese a structured meal plan along with instructions to "quit eating too much." The most successful popular diet books are those that promise rapid weight loss by altering the type of foods to be eaten.

In contrast, behavioral programs have focused on *how* to eat. An individual is to control weight by controlling the environmental events that precipitate overeating. Eating patterns are to change as patients are instructed to slow the rate of eating, alter the stimulus environment so food is not available, reward new eating habits, increase energy expenditure, and monitor eating behaviors as well as food intake. Very little mention is made of food, although about a 1200-calorie diet is usually nested in these programs.

The research that has resulted from this approach has focused on the development of techniques designed to alter eating behaviors (for example, whether to monitor food intake before or after a meal). The relative efficacy of behavioral programs suggests that conceptualizing eating disorders in this fashion is worthwhile. Yet weight losses have been consistent in behavioral studies and have not been clinically significant. In addition, long-term weight loss is very unusual. A new conceptual approach may be useful.

Perhaps the major question should change from what behaviors to prescribe to how to adhere to prescribed behaviors. The basic prescription for weight loss is simple—eat less and exercise more. The behavioral techniques may be helpful at encouraging these behaviors for a short time, but the almost universal relapse that occurs within the first year after treatment suggests that more needs to be done. In retrospect, it is easy to see that people with a lifelong history of overeating cannot achieve long-term weight loss with a 10- or 12-week program that proposes new eating behaviors. The high attrition rates in most studies show that patients have difficulty staying with any program long enough to attain ideal weight. I suggest that the principles of behavior be applied to the issue of adherence: how well people comply with prescribed behaviors in existing programs.

Adherence to exercise. Despite its benefits, exercise is useful only to the extent it is undertaken. Exercise is not popular among people in general and even less so among the obese. Attrition rates from exercise programs average 50 percent, even in the case of motivated patients who are recovering from myocardial infarction (cf. Brownell & Stunkard, 1980). With obese women, Gwinup (1975) found that only 32 percent completed a one-year program requiring only modest activity (walking).

Alternate exercise habits. For the purpose of considering the adherence issue, it may be useful to conceptualize activity in two categories: programmed and life-style activity. Programmed activity consists of regularly scheduled bouts of activities usually thought to be "exercise." These include running, calisthenics, swimming, cycling, taking part in regular sporting events, and so forth. That these activities are beneficial is indisputable. Whether obese people will do them is another matter. Two studies have used behavioral procedures, particularly contracting, to increase adherence to exercise programs (Epstein, Thompson, & Wing, 1980; Wysocki, Hall, Iwata, & Riordan, 1979). These results are very encouraging, but poor adherence to exercise programs among the obese makes life-style programs seem like an attractive alternative.

Life-style activities are those that can be worked into day-to-day patterns of living. These might include parking a car some distance from one's destination to increase walking, standing rather than sitting, and generally increasing movement throughout the day. One such method is using stairs rather than elevators or escalators (Brownell, Stunkard, & Albaum, 1980). Climbing stairs requires greater energy expenditure per unit time than almost any other activity, it is one of the few activities related to decreased risk of heart disease (Paffenbarger, Wing, & Hyde, 1978), and it holds the promise of adherence over the long term. Many behaviors are available for increasing life-style exercise (Brownell, 1980), but, as yet, no studies are available to determine whether programmed or life-style activities are most beneficial.

Attitude Restructuring

The feelings and attitudes held by obese persons about their bodies, their self-control, their past dieting efforts, their prognosis for success, and their ability to control their lives can influence their ability to lose weight. For example, a dieter may eat ice cream even though it is "fattening." The response, although it may not be clearly articulated in the dieter's mind, may be, "I have no willpower," or "This proves I will be fat forever," or "I am disgusting because I have no control." The feelings that result from this self-statement (guilt, depression, anxiety) are likely to undermine the dieter's resolve when the next eating episode occurs. Mahoney and Mahoney (1976a) have presented many of the maladaptive cognitions that dieters experience, along with means of establishing new attitudes.

Countering self-defeating thoughts can be difficult and requires great persistence by both the professional and the patient. Identification of these attitudes can be aided by knowing the categories into which they fall and by providing the patients with rational alternatives to their inappropriate thoughts. Table 4.1, adapted from Brownell (1980), gives possible categories for self-defeating attitudes and possible restatements.

In the past several years, new methods for behavioral treatment have yielded very encouraging findings. These have been presented in detail in a recent review (Stunkard & Brownell, 1979). However, the approaches with the greatest promise and greatest likelihood of influencing program adherence have involved intervention into the social environment. Interventions of this sort may also be relevant to other substance-abuse areas.

Modifying the Social Environment

Eating and exercise behaviors, and obesity itself, do not occur in a social vacuum. People in general, including the obese, are responsive to family, friends, people in the work environment, fraternal and religious groups, self-help groups, and so forth. It may be possible to exploit or even modify these naturally occurring social events to en-

Table 4.1. Categories of Self-defeating Attitudes and Examples of Rational Restatements

Attitude Category	Rational Restatement
Light Bulb Thinking	
Example: "Now that I ate that cake, I am off the diet and I may as well give up and let go."	"There's nothing wrong with the cake as long as my calories are in check. I can always cut back later."
The Impossible Dream	
Example: "No more potato chips for me. I'll just have celery and carrot sticks from now on."	"I know I love potato chips and if I have some once in a while, it won't hurt me. This way, I'll get to enjoy the foods I like."
Imperatives	
Example: "I'll *never* eat ice cream again and I'll exercise *every* day."	"I can't expect myself to be perfect, so I'll do the best I can. Even if I only exercise sometimes and do eat ice cream occasionally, I am far better off than when I started."
Dead End Thinking	
Example: "I have no willpower and I just can't resist temptation."	"I'm making progress all the time, and I can't expect to be rid of lifelong problems in a few weeks."
Wishful Thinking	
Example: "Thin people have it made. They don't know how lucky they are."	"Thin people have their problems too, and they may even be worse than mine."

courage long-term adherence to dietary regimens. The three areas that have received the most attention are the family, the work site, and community self-help groups. Information on work-site programs can also be obtained in other papers (Foreyt, Scott, & Gotto, 1980; Stunkard & Brownell, 1980) and self-help groups have been reviewed by Stunkard and Brownell (1979).

Family Intervention–Couples Training

Eating is a social event for most people, and the family may be the source of many social interactions involving food. Someone in the family must purchase, prepare, and serve the meals. The family is a natural source of social influence. Several researchers have studied the importance of this effect on eating.

Stuart (reported in Stuart & Davis, 1972) tape recorded and scored mealtime interactions between 14 overweight women and their husbands. They found that (1) husbands were seven times more likely than their weight-reducing wives to initiate food-relevant topics of conversation; (2) husbands were almost four times as likely as their wives to proffer food to the spouse; (3) wives were slightly over twice as likely as their husbands to reject food offers; and (4) husbands were over twelve times as likely to offer criticism of their wives' eating behavior as they were to praise it. Stuart and Davis (1972) maintain that some spouses " . . . are not only not contributors to their wives' efforts to lose weight, but they may actually exert a negative influence" (pp. 19–20).

Mahoney and Mahoney (1976b) evaluated "social support engineering" as one component of a treatment program for obese subjects. A social support index was calculated based on attendance and therapists' reports of family cooperation. The correlations between the social-support index and treatment outcome were 0.92 at posttreatment, 0.33 at six months, 0.34 at one year, and 0.63 at two years. Although the involvement of family members had been touted as a facilitative factor in weight control (Mahoney & Mahoney, 1976b; O'Leary & Wilson, 1975; Stuart & Davis, 1972), no direct studies of family intervention had been done.

In the first study to systematically manipulate and evaluate the influence of family intervention, Wilson and Brownell (1978) assigned obese subjects to either family-member-present or family-member-absent conditions. In the family-member-absent groups, subjects received the standard behavioral program described by Stuart and Davis (1972). In the family-member-present condition, subjects received the same program but were also required to attend all sessions with a family member in order to (1) acquaint family members with the principles of behavioral weight control treatments; (2) instruct them to cease criticizing their partner's weight and eating behaviors; (3) teach them to reinforce improved eating habits; and (4) instruct them to assist their partners' attempts to restructure the conditions and consequences of overeating. After an eight-week treatment phase and a six-month follow-up, there were no differences in the amount of weight lost between persons assigned to the two conditions. The authors concluded that the failure of the family intervention may have resulted from a lack of structure for the family members' behavior, and from the fact that some of the family members were not exerting a powerful enough social influence (some were sisters, daughters, and so forth).

A subsequent study by Brownell, Heckerman, Westlake, Hayes, & Monti (1978b) evaluated the involvement of spouses in the treatment process. In this program, the couple rather than the individual was the focus of treatment. Subjects and spouses were instructed in a variety of behavioral techniques including mutual monitoring of food-related behaviors, stimulus control, modeling, and reinforcement. For each part of the patients' program there was a corresponding part for the spouses, who participated fully in each training session. Subjects were given a manual that described a ten-week sequence of behavioral techniques, and spouses were given their own manual to underscore the need for behavior change for both subjects and spouses. The spouses were taught to model appropriate eating behaviors such as slowing the rate of eating and eating in particular locations to "set a good example." Similarly, they were instructed in stimulus control so that they would avoid exposing the subjects to food cues and were encouraged to engage the subject during times of temptation in activities incompatible with eating. Each partner monitored the other partner's behavior as well as his or her own. The program stressed that mutual effort was critical to success.

This couples program was compared to two other experimental conditions. In one condition, dieters had "cooperative" spouses who had agreed to take part in the couples program, but the dieters were treated alone. In the other condition, dieters had "noncooperative" spouses who refused to participate. Treatment sessions were held weekly for ten weeks, with monthly booster sessions following for six months. Figure 4.1 shows the superiority of the couples training group. At the end of treatment, the couples group had lost 20 pounds, the "cooperative spouse—subject alone" condition had lost 15 pounds, and the "noncooperative spouse" condition had lost 12 pounds. These weight losses did not differ statistically, but after the six-month maintenance phase, the couples group had increased their mean weight loss to 30 pounds—significantly more than the other two conditions (19 and 15 pounds, respectively). These findings were noteworthy because the weight losses during treatment were nearly triple those reported in other studies on behavior therapy, and because one-third of the total weight loss in the couples condition occurred *after* active treatment ended.

The study by Brownell and colleagues (1978b) was followed by several others on couples training, family intervention, or involving friends in the treatment program. In total, five studies found a beneficial effect for social environment interventions (Brownell et al., 1978b; Fremouw & Zitter, 1980; Israel & Saccone, 1979; Pearce, LeBow, &

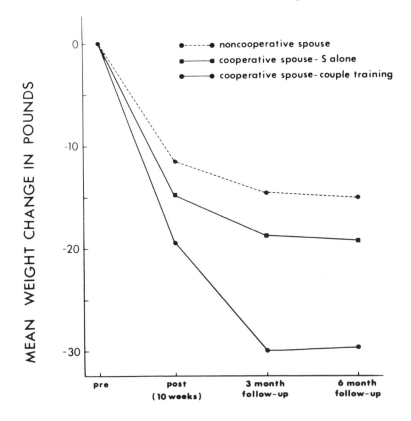

TIME OF ASSESSMENT

Figure 4.1. Mean weight change in pounds for three conditions of spouse intervention.

Reprinted with permission from *Behaviour Research and Therapy,* Vol. 16, Brownell, K. D., Heckerman, C. L., Westlake, R. J., Hayes, S. C., & Monti, P. M., The effect of couples training and partner cooperativeness in the behavioral treatment of obesity. Copyright © 1978, Pergamon Press, Ltd.

Orchard, 1979; Rosenthal, Allen, & Winter, 1980). Three other studies did not find this effect (O'Neil, Currey, Hirsch, Riddle, Taylor, Malcolm, & Sexauer, 1979; Wilson & Brownell, 1978; Zitter & Fremouw, 1978). One factor that distinguished effective from ineffective programs was whether the social-support partners played an active role in treatment. It appeared that active participation by cooperative spouses could facilitate weight loss and the maintenance of that loss.

Work-Site Intervention

A second forum for mobilizing social influence is the work site. Millions of people spend much of their day at a place of employment. Patterns of interaction develop among workers and between employees and employers. This naturally occurring social system has many advantages as a means for health-behavior changes. Time away from work is kept to a minimum—an hour each week for 20 weeks may be sufficient for many life-style change programs. The work site can provide space and clerical staff to support a program. The employer and fellow employees of an individual can exert strong sanctions for attendance—a luxury not available in most leisure-time programs. The increased morale that may develop from cooperation or competition between groups at the work site may increase treatment efficacy. Such a program is a worthy investment for any industry that pays the health care costs for its employees. Health improvement can easily repay the costs of such programs through decreased absenteeism, improved work performance, decreased hospitalization, and more intangible factors like improved morale (Stunkard, 1981).

A work-site intervention program for the treatment of hypertension has shown the value of this approach. In this program, members of the United Store Workers Union in New York City took part in a hypertension-control program at the Gimbels and Bloomingdale's stores (Alderman, 1976; Alderman & Schoenbaum, 1975). Before the program, less than half of the hypertensive union members had achieved blood pressure control, and those who subsequently refused entry into the program continued at about this level of control. When the program began, blood pressure screening was done at the stores by nurse practitioners. Hypertensive persons were then seen by a physician and medication was prescribed, if necessary. Periodic meetings were scheduled and members were encouraged to attend through postcard reminders and calls from a union employee. Participants carried cards that showed their blood pressures and were awarded a certificate when blood pressure control was achieved. This work-site program resulted in blood pressure control in 80 percent of the participants and radically reduced days of hospitalization for cardiovascular disease.

This program stands in contrast to another work-site program conducted in Canada for hypertensive foundry workers (Sackett, Gibson, Taylor, Haynes, Hackett, Roberts, & Johnson, 1975). Participants were offered blood pressure treatment and screening but were not part of the same social influence system as outlined above. The *esprit de corps* engendered by the union support was lacking, and there were no rewards for adherence to the scheduled meetings. Blood pressure control occurred in only 50 percent of the foundry workers.

It appears, therefore, that the work site is an ideal location for a weight-reduction program or for other programs that encourage health-behavior changes (for example, smoking reduction). However, the manner in which the program is administered can be a critical factor. Social influence factors that operate at a work site can be quite powerful, and a program must be designed to take full advantage of these factors.

In collaboration with Dr. Albert J. Stunkard, I am conducting a work-site intervention program for weight reduction at the United Store Workers Union. A pilot program has been completed at one Gimbels store and has yielded promising results. We are experimenting with training union members to serve as group leaders and with holding sessions at different times of day and at different intervals.

The Community as a Social System

The community itself is another naturally occurring social system with unique patterns of interaction among its members. Until recently it was thought that to allow for experimental control in a study of health interventions, members of a community should be randomized among treatment conditions. This, however, may dissipate the very social influence that could make a community intervention effective. It may be more fruitful to use entire communities as experimental groups and randomize interventions among communities (Stunkard, 1981). The Stanford Heart Disease Prevention Program is an example of this (Farquhar et al., 1977).

In the Stanford program, large-scale interventions were used to reduce cardiovascular risk factors (Farquhar et al., 1977; Maccoby, Farquhar, Wood, & Alexander, 1977). An intensive and sophisticated two-year campaign in this three-community study included three hours of television programs; 50 television spots; 100 radio spots; several hours of radio programming; weekly newspaper columns; newspaper stories and advertisements; posters used in buses, stores, and work sites; and printed materials mailed directly to participants. Three communities in northern California were used. The population of each was about 14,000. One town received the media campaign, and another served as a control and received no campaign. In the third community, the media campaign was supplemented by a face-to-face behavioral instruction program directed at two-thirds of the participants identified as being in the upper 25 percent of those at risk for coronary heart disease.

The results were most promising. After the second year of the campaign, the risk of coronary heart disease had decreased 17 percent in the treatment communities, whereas the risk had increased 6 percent in the control community. In the treatment communities, there were reductions in cholesterol levels, smoking, and blood pressure. It is interesting that the media campaign and the face-to-face instruction had significant effects on all variables except relative weight. It is possible that more structured and intensive interventions are needed to supplement a media campaign if weight reduction is to occur.

The Stanford three-community study is informative for several reasons. First, it shows that media campaigns designed to reach large numbers of persons can be effective at changing some health-related behaviors. The long-term maintenance of these changes has yet to be studied, but initial change is possible. Second, the media campaign may be effective in prompting people who need additional instruction to seek such assistance. Third, it may be possible to utilize the social pressures of a community and still maintain experimental control by testing an intervention on an entire community and using another community as a control. Fourth, specific behavioral instruction may be necessary for a health education program to be effective; disease information may not be sufficient.

Conclusion

Obesity may serve as a useful focal point for discussions of substance abuse, including smoking, alcoholism, and drug abuse. Because the dependent variable, weight, is so easily measured, obesity has served as a proving ground for countless behavioral and nonbehavioral strategies. The result has been a dramatic increase in our knowledge of the principles of behavior in general and in our ability to treat the obese in particular.

Behavioral interventions have been reasonably effective at producing short-term weight change. Controlled research has shown that behavior therapy is more effective than any treatment approach to which it has been compared. Early studies failed to include long-term follow-up, and therefore there were enthusiastic claims of the potency of behavior therapy for the obese. As the long-term results become available, it appears that permanent weight control is something of a wish rather than a reality. Relapse, which plagues all areas of substance abuse, is a particular problem for the obese, because repeated weight loss followed by weight gain may be more dangerous than static obesity. Research on animals and humans has shown that repeated episodes of dieting can be associated with cardiovascular problems and psychological distress (Brownell, 1978).

The lack of long-term efficacy is not cause to abandon the behavioral approach. Initial behavior change and the maintenance of that change may be governed by different processes (Bandura, 1969; Kazdin & Wilson, 1978). Behavior therapy studies for the most part have focused on initial behavior change and have been relatively successful. It is time for more research into the critical issue of maintenance. More specifically, why do so many people drop out of treatment, and of those who remain in treatment, why do so few adhere to program directives?

Conceptualizing the treatment of obesity as an adherence problem may lead to new ideas for research. Behavioral principles have been used almost exclusively for the modification of eating behaviors. Little effort has been devoted to testing methods of improving adherence to these eating-behavior regimens. Implementing strong monetary contracts for caloric restriction or weight loss may be effective (Jeffery, Thompson, & Wing, 1977). Altering the schedule of treatment meetings may also be useful; the most frequent contact could occur during the difficult maintenance period, rather than at the outset of a treatment program, when most people are strongly motivated. But the most promising approach to date is the modification of the social environment.

For any person there are a number of naturally occurring social environments that can exert a powerful influence on behavior. The three major social environments are home, work site, and community. Studies in each of the areas have been very encouraging, although the data are preliminary at best. Intervening in the social environment allows mobilization of social forces that may be much more powerful than the impact of treatment sessions scheduled once each week. This pervasive influence may lead to improved adherence to prescribed behaviors because of important sources of reinforcement that are available many times each day, and because of an increase in the number of discriminative stimuli that prompt appropriate behaviors.

References

Alderman, M. H. Organization for long-term management of hypertension. *Bulletin of the New York Academy of Medicine,* 1976, *52,* 697–717.

Alderman, M. H., & Schoenbaum, E. E. Detection and treatment of hypertension at the work site. *New England Journal of Medicine,* 1975, *293,* 65–68.

Ashby, W. A., & Wilson, G. T. Behavior therapy for obesity: Booster sessions and long-term maintenance of weight loss. *Behavior Research and Therapy,* 1977, *15,* 451–464.

Bandura, A. *Principles of behavior modification.* New York: Holt, Rinehart, and Winston, 1969.

Bandura, A., & Simon, K. M. The role of proximal intentions in self-regulation of refractory behavior. *Cognitive Therapy Research,* 1977, *1,* 177–193.

Brownell, K. D. The psychological and medical sequelae of nonprescription weight reduction programs. Paper presented at the Annual Meeting of the American Psychological Association, Toronto, August, 1978.

Brownell, K. D. *The partnership diet program.* New York: Rawson-Wade, 1980.

Brownell, K. D., Heckerman, C. L., & Westlake, R. J. The behavioral control of obesity: A descriptive analysis of a large-scale program. Unpublished manuscript, Brown University, 1976.

Brownell, K. D., Heckerman, C. L., & Westlake, R. J. Therapist and group contact as variables in the behavioral treatment of obesity. *Journal of Consulting and Clinical Psychology,* 1978, *46,* 593–594. (a)

Brownell, K. D., Heckerman, C. L., Westlake, R. J., Hayes, S. C., & Monti, P. M. The effect of couples training and partner cooperativeness in the behavioral treatment of obesity. *Behavior Research and Therapy,* 1978, *16,* 323–333. (b)

Brownell, K. D., & Stunkard, A. J. Exercise in the development and control of obesity. In A. J. Stunkard (Ed.), *Obesity.* Philadelphia: Saunders, 1980.

Brownell, K. D., Stunkard, A. J., & Albaum, J. M. Evaluation and modification of exercise patterns in the natural environment. *American Journal of Psychiatry,* 1980, *137,* 1540–1545.

Build and blood pressure study. Chicago: Society of Actuaries, 1959.

Diament, C., & Wilson, G. T. An experimental investigation of the effects of covert sensitization in an analogue eating situation. *Behavior Therapy,* 1975, *6,* 499–509.

Epstein, L. H., Thompson, J. K., & Wing, R. R. The effects of contract and lottery procedures on attendance and fitness in aerobics exercise. *Behavior Modification,* 1980, *4,* 465–480.

Farquhar, J. W., Maccoby, N., Wood, P. D., Alexander, J. K., Breitrose, H., Brown, B. W., Haskell, W. L., McAlister, A. L., Meyer, A. J., Nash, J. D., & Stern, M. P. Community education for cardiovascular health. *Lancet,* 1977, *1,* 1192–1195.

Fernan, W. S. The role of experimenter contact in behavioral bibliotherapy of obesity. Unpublished manuscript, Pennsylvania State University, 1973.

Ferstl, R., Jokusch, V., & Brengelman, J. C. Die verhaltenstherapeutische Behandlung des Übergewichts. *International Journal of Health Education,* 1975, *18,* 119–136.

Foreyt, J. P., & Hagen, R. L. Covert sensitization: Conditioning or suggestion? *Journal of Abnormal Psychology,* 1973, *82,* 17–23.

Foreyt, J. P., & Kennedy, W. A. Treatment of overweight by aversion therapy. *Behavior Research and Therapy,* 1971, *9,* 29–34.

Foreyt, J. P., Scott, L. W., & Gotto, A. M. Weight control and nutrition education programs in occupational settings. *Public Health Reports,* 1980, *95,* 127–136.

Fremouw, W. J., & Zitter, R. E. Individual and couple behavioral contracting for weight reduction and maintenance. *Behavior Therapist,* 1980, *3,* 15–16.

Goldblatt, P. B., Moore, M. E., & Stunkard, A. J. Social factors in obesity. *Journal of the American Medical Association,* 1965, *192,* 1039–1044.

Gordon, T., & Kannel, W. B. Obesity and cardiovascular disease: The Framingham Study. *Journal of Clinical Endocrinology and Metabolism,* 1976, *5,* 367–375.

Green, L. Temporal and stimulus factors in self-monitoring by obese persons. *Behavior Therapy,* 1978, *9,* 328–341.

Gwinup, G. Effect of exercise alone on the weight of obese women. *Archives of Internal Medicine,* 1975, *135,* 676–680.

Hagen, R. L. Group therapy versus bibliotherapy in weight reduction. *Behavior Therapy,* 1974, *5,* 222–234.

Hanson, R. W., Borden, B. L., Hall, S. M., & Hall, R. G. Use of programmed instruction in teaching self-management skills to overweight adults. *Behavior Therapy,* 1976, *7,* 366–373.

Harris, M. B. Self-directed program for weight control: A pilot study. *Journal of Abnormal Psychology,* 1969, *74,* 263–270.

Harris, M. B., & Hallbauer, E. S. Self-directed weight control through eating and exercise. *Behavior Research and Therapy,* 1973, *11,* 523–529.

Health and Nutrition Survey. Height and weight of adults 18–74 years of age in the United States. National Center for Health Statistics. *Advance Data from Vital Health Statistics,* No. 3, pp. 1–18, November 19, 1976.

Israel, A. C., & Saccone, A. J. Follow-up effects of choice of mediator and target of reinforcement on weight loss. Behavior Therapy, 1979, *10,* 260–265.

Jeffery, R. W., Thompson, P. D., & Wing, R. R. Effects on weight reduction of strong monetary contracts for calorie restriction or weight loss. Unpublished manuscript, Stanford University, 1977.

Jeffery, R. W., Wing, R. R., & Stunkard, A. J. Behavioral treatment of obesity: The state of the art in 1976. *Behavior Therapy,* 1978, *9,* 189–199.

Kannel, W. B., & Gordon, T. Risks and hazards of obesity. Paper presented at the Fogarty Conference on Obesity, Washington, D. C., 1979.

Kazdin, A. E., & Wilson, G. T. *Evaluation of behavior therapy: Issues, evidence, and research strategies.* Cambridge, Mass.: Ballinger, 1978.

Kingsley, R. G., & Wilson, G. T. Behavior therapy for obesity: A comparative investigation of long-term efficacy. *Journal of Consulting and Clinical Psychology*, 1977, *45*, 288–298.

Maccoby, N., Farquhar, J. W., Wood, P. D., & Alexander, J. Reducing the risk of cardiovascular disease: Effects of a community-based campaign on knowledge and behavior. *Journal of Community Health*, 1977, *3*, 100–114.

Mahoney, M. J. Self-reward and self-monitoring techniques for weight control. *Behavior Therapy*, 1974, *5*, 48–57.

Mahoney, M. J., & Mahoney, K. *Permanent weight control: A total solution to the dieter's dilemma.* New York: Norton, 1976. (a)

Mahoney, M. J., & Mahoney, K. Treatment of obesity: A clinical exploration. In B. J. Williams, S. Martin, & J. P. Foreyt (Eds.), *Obesity: Behavioral approaches to dietary management.* New York: Brunner/Mazel, 1976. (b)

Mann, G. V. The influence of obesity on health. *New England Journal of Medicine*, 1974, *291*, 178–185, 226–232.

Metropolitan Life Insurance Company. Frequency of overweight and underweight. *Statistical Bulletin of the Metropolitan Life Insurance Company*, 1960, *41*, 4–7.

O'Leary, K. D., & Wilson, G. T. *Behavior therapy: Applications and outcome.* Englewood Cliffs, N.J.: Prentice-Hall, 1975.

O'Neil, P. M., Currey, H. S., Hirsch, A. A., Riddle, F. E., Taylor, C. I., Malcolm, R. J., & Sexauer, J. D. Effects of sex of subject and spouse involvement on weight loss in a behavioral treatment program: A retrospective investigation. *Addictive Behaviors*, 1979, *4*, 167–178.

Paffenbarger, R. S., Wing, A. L., & Hyde, R. T. Physical activity as an index of heart attack risk in college alumni. *American Journal of Epidemiology*, 1978, *108*, 161–175.

Pearce, J. W., LeBow, M. D., & Orchard, J. The role of spouse involvement in the behavioral treatment of obese women. Paper presented at the annual meeting of the Canadian Psychological Association, Quebec, 1979.

Penick, S. B., Filion, R., Fox, S., & Stunkard, A. J. Behavior modification in the treatment of obesity. *Psychosomatic Medicine*, 1971, *33*, 49–55.

Romanczyk, R. G. Self-monitoring in the treatment of obesity: Parameters of reactivity. *Behavior Therapy*, 1974, *5*, 531–540.

Romanczyk, R. G., Tracey, D. A., Wilson, G. T., & Thorpe, G. L. Behavioral techniques in the treatment of obesity: A comparative analysis. *Behavioral Research and Therapy*, 1973, *11*, 629–640.

Rosenthal, B., Allen, G. J., & Winter, C. Husband involvement in the behavioral treatment of overweight women: Initial effects and long-term follow-up. *International Journal of Obesity*, 1980, *4*, 165–173.

Sackett, D. L., Gibson, E. S., Taylor, D. W., Haynes, B. R., Hackett, B. C., Roberts, R. S., & Johnson, A. L. Randomized clinical trial of strategies for improving medication compliance in primary hypertension. *Lancet*, 1975, *31*, 1205–1207.

Stalonas, P. M., Johnson, W. G., & Christ, M. Behavior modification for obesity: The evaluation of exercise, contingency management, and program adherence. *Journal of Consulting and Clinical Psychology*, 1978, *46*, 463–469.

Stuart, R. B. Behavioral control of overeating. *Behavior Research and Therapy*, 1967, *5*, 357–365.

Stuart, R. B., & Davis, B. *Slim chance in a fat world: Behavioral Control of Obesity.* Champaign, Ill.: Research Press, 1972.

Stunkard, A. J. The management of obesity. *New York State Journal of Medicine*, 1958, *58*, 79–87.

Stunkard, A. J. From explanation to action in psychosomatic medicine: The case of obesity. *Psychosomatic Medicine*, 1975, *37*, 195–236.

Stunkard, A. J. The practice of health promotion: The case of obesity. In L. Ng & D. Davis (Eds.), *Strategies for public health: Promoting health and preventing disease.* New York: Van Nostrand Reinhold, 1981, pp. 297–316.

Stunkard, A. J., & Brownell, K. D. Behavior therapy and self-help programs for obesity. In J. F. Munro (Ed.), *The treatment of obesity.* London, MIP Press, 1979.

Stunkard, A. J., & Brownell, K. D. Work site treatment for obesity. *American Journal of Psychiatry*, 1980, *137*, 252–253.

Stunkard, A. J., & McLaren-Hume, M. The results of treatment for obesity. *Archives of Internal Medicine*, 1959, *103*, 79–85.

Stunkard, A. J., & Penick, S. B. Behavior modification in the treatment of obesity: The problem of maintaining weight loss. *Archives of General Psychiatry*, 1979, *36*, 801–806.

Stunkard, A. J., & Rush, A. J. Dieting and depression reexamined: A critical review of reports of untoward responses during weight reduction for obesity. *Annals of Internal Medicine*, 1974, *81*, 526–533.

U.S. Department of Health, Education and Welfare. Public Health Service. *Obesity and health.* Washington, D. C., U.S. Government Printing Office, 1966.

Van Itallie, T. B. Testimony before Senate Select Committee on Nutrition and Human Needs. Washington, D. C., U.S. Government Printing Office, 1977.

Waxler, S. H., & Leef, M. F. Obesity—Doctor's dilemma. *Geriatrics*, 1969, *24*, 98–108.

Wilson, G. T., & Brownell, K. D. Behavior therapy for obesity: Including family members in the treatment process. *Behavior Therapy*, 1978, *9*, 943–945.

Wollersheim, J. P. Effectiveness of group therapy based on learning principles in the treatment of overweight women. *Journal of Abnormal Psychology*, 1970, *76*, 462–474.

Wysocki, T., Hall, G., Iwata, B., & Riordan, M. Behavioral management of exercise: Contracting for aerobic points. *Journal of Applied Behavior Analysis*, 1979, *12*, 55–64.

Zitter, R. E., & Fremouw, W. J. Individual versus partner consequation for weight loss. *Behavior Therapy*, 1978, *9*, 808–813.

5

Treatment and Outcome in Anorexia Nervosa

Arthur H. Crisp

In order to evaluate the outcome of treatment in anorexia nervosa one must, of course, first satisfactorily define "outcome," "treatment," and "anorexia nervosa," and then conduct an appropriately designed study involving random allocation of such "patients" to the general or specific treatment/no-treatment experience. If "outcome" is defined as anything other than just immediate and slight weight gain then there is no such study reported in the literature. Most major follow-up studies used measures of body weight, eating behavior, reproductive function, and sexual and social adjustment and have defined "recovery" in terms of the individual's close approximation to normality in all these respects. Such follow-up studies, some more thorough and detailed than others, have been widely reported over the past 20 years. Although within them some or all of the "patients" have sometimes received "treatment," there has been no means of evaluating its impact. Nor is it certain that the patient groups were similar in the various studies except that they all had what is widely accepted as "anorexia nervosa." Indeed, recent studies have demonstrated certain clinical features associated with poor prognosis, and these may well have been differently represented in the various groups of patients studied and reported. It is not always possible, from the reports, even to determine whether the severity of the disorder was similar or not in the different groups.

Under these circumstances I shall concern myself mainly with a review of my own opinions about the nature and evolution of anorexia nervosa, the nature of our treatment approach, and, so far as I can, a judgment of its short- and long-term effects.

The Nature and Evolution of Anorexia Nervosa

Figure 5.1 shows, in diagrammatic form, some aspects of the evolution of anorexia nervosa. The emphasis is upon the pivotal significance of puberty and the phobic avoidance stance within the condition. The threshold weights reflect significant stages of sexual maturation within the pubertal processes around which the disorder pivots. Established anorexia nervosa is rooted in the need to maintain body weight and shape below this threshold—a task that demands maintenance of what is inherently biologically a most unstable position and constantly subject to the natural thrust of early pubertal growth and related appetite. In the face of this constant threat of weight gain through the threshold, the anorectic retreats into increasingly low body weight and becomes ever more terrified of any slight weight gain reflecting and revealing to others her loss of control over the situation. Only if she has absolute control over the maintenance of her body weight at a barely subpubertal level, for which the mechanism of freely vomiting usually needs to

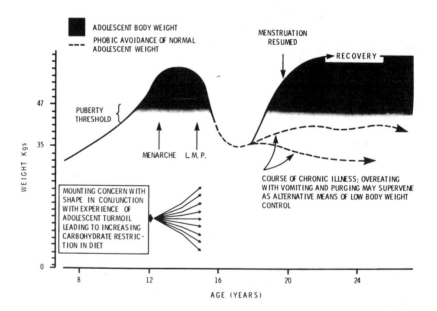

Figure 5.1.   The evolution of anorexia nervosa is shown in diagrammatic form in this figure. The threshold weights are shown in representative form.

Reproduced with permission from Crisp, A. H. *Anorexia nervosa: Let me be.* London: Academic Press, 1980. Copyright © by Academic Press, Inc. (London) Ltd.

be available, may she then honestly claim that, indeed, she does not wish to lose more weight. Under these circumstances her adult body weight phobia and associated avoidance behavior will be even more rigorously denied than usual, revealed only in a situation in which she loses the freedom to sustain her current delicate weight-control mechanisms.

The anorectic shows the same desperate need to control and manipulate her or his environment as does the "hysteric" in order to protect their fragile social adjustment. The avoidance stance, in relation to biologically mature body weight, reflects her condensed terror of its social consequences and her inability to handle these difficulties in any less primitive (e.g., neurotic) way. Low body weight control may be sustained mainly by carbohydrate avoidance, a form of "starvation" unique to anorexia nervosa, or else by the binging/vomiting/purging syndrome, which confers a very different metabolic stance but which is nevertheless still subpubertal though less stably so. This latter stance is significantly associated with premorbid impulsivity, especially in respect to eating and sexual behavior. It is a feature of the chronic condition, sometimes also being associated with behavior such as shoplifting, and it leads to complications such as epilepsy, periodic edema, severe abdominal discomfort, and gastric dilatation and is more likely than other variants of the condition to lead to premature death by either suicide or profound metabolic decompensation. Other factors associated with poor prognosis include late age of onset, poor childhood adjustment, impaired parental, marital, and personal psychosocial adjustments, lower social class background, and probably also premorbid borderline personality structure and being male.

In the natural course of events approximately 40 percent of individuals with severe anorexia nervosa will be found recovered six years after initial accurate clinic screening, and about 5 percent will be dead. However, there are probably a number of anorectics who avoid medical attention altogether and others who linger, misdiagnosed, in a variety of clinics. These latter groups may evolve differently; we do not know.

Treatment Approach

In the first instance I shall describe briefly our treatment approach, established now for 20 years and within which we have experience of over 300 anorectics treated on an initial inpatient basis involving, as part of the program, restoration of body weight back to matched population mean levels (Crisp, 1967, 1977, 1980). As can be seen in Figure 5.2, mean body weight increases under these circumstances from 38 kg to 54 kg on average. It is obvious that no anorectic would persist in such a circumstance if she were simply and in isolation to experience this as *being done to her*. For success to be possible the anorectic needs to be identified with the process. The treatment approach is based on the premise that (1) the disorder is rooted in a phobic avoidance mechanism; (2) that the thing being avoided is adult body weight, which is seen by the anorectic as alien, inflicted from without, and terrifying; (3) that this weight has in the past presented overwhelming psychosocial challenges to the anorectic and her family; and (4) that the anorectic may so far have little in the way of more sophisticated potential social coping devices available within her.

Anorectics see their state as egosyntonic. For them it is socially adaptive. Others wishing to change them must aspire to help them

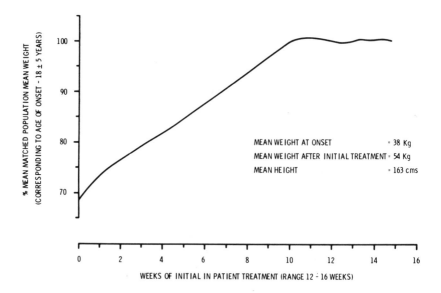

Figure 5.2. The immediate effect of inpatient treatment on body weight in just over 300 patients severely ill with anorexia nervosa, who underwent this phase of care, 1960–1978 (excluding nine patients who discharged themselves during the process).

Reproduced with permission from Crisp, A. H. *Anorexia nervosa: Let me be.* London: Academic Press, 1980. Copyright © by Academic Press, Inc. (London) Ltd.

become "patients"—people feeling themselves afflicted with the disorder that they hope those others will be able to help them shed.

I believe that adolescent maturational challenges reflect family and wider social dynamics impinging on the former's development and ultimately upon the experiences promoting the anorexia nervosa itself. They are the same challenges that others, more resourceful, might cope with or otherwise respond to by falling ill in other ways, depending on their own and their families' biological and psychosocial makeup. If an anorectic is to be helped to grapple with this challenge then she must (1) enter the arena once more, that is, achieve normal adult body weight, and (2) develop other coping mechanisms. Neither step can be achieved easily without the other, and the second step will be much easier if she is not long established in her anorexia nervosa and if changes are also possible within the family. This will require positive shifts of attitude rather than any further manipulation such as crudely separating the anorectic from her family. Elsewhere I have recently again described in detail our initial approach to the anorectic family (Crisp, 1980). We strive to engage all parents (and occasionally spouses and others) in treatment and succeed in about 85 percent of instances. In other cases parents are dead, too geographically remote from us, or, very occasionally, too hostile for this to happen. Not all parents by any means have a globally brittle personal or marital adjustment. In one way or another the maturation of this particular offspring has challenged them, exposed their Achilles' heel. In the initial outpatient consultation this dynamic needs to be identified, and we strive routinely to achieve this before we have even met the anorectic. The subsequent encounter with the anorectic will be enriched by such knowledge and this, combined with some understanding that the clinician has of the psychological mechanisms at work within anorexia nervosa, can be used to advantage in attempting to gain the anorectic's trust from the outset. The anorectic will need to come to terms with the dual nature of any subsequent treatment and will initially be terrified at the prospect of the major weight gain. Trapped into this constellation, she will have been envisaging at the most some small weight gain up to an immediate subpubertal level, say 40 kg. She can be assured that, though in bed, eating a normal diet, and gaining weight at the rate of 1½ kg a week, (1) she will be protected from overeating; (2) no one is going to tell her that she "looks well" when she has gained the weight (on the contrary all staff will recognize that, at this stage, she feels more sustainedly chaotic, terrified, and despairing than ever); and (3) she will be involved in intensive psychotherapy directed at her need to cope first and foremost with her refound adult body shape; the need for

herself and others to come to see her as more than merely this body
shape; and her need to develop new coping resources.

This initial inpatient program lasts about four months and allows,
apart from the weight gain, the establishment of important
psychotherapeutic relationships and friendship with the individual
and the family through the mechanisms of individual, family, group,
and milieu psychotherapy. Early interpretation of the transference can
be crucially important in order to allow the anorectic to explore the
new environment. All staff seek to befriend the patient during this
period, allowing a rich range of potentially healthy identifications. The
parents are included in this milieu approach.

Family psychotherapy usually focuses first on the parents, who will
sometimes themselves be seen individually for awhile to allow further
identification of their personal past experiences, needs, and attitudes.
The bringing together of the parents and, later on, the patient can then
optimally facilitate the sharing of experiences, especially adolescent
experiences of all its members together with feelings past and present.
Powerfully enmeshed families will themselves often expose the pathological nature of their bonding. Apathetic and defective parents can
sometimes declare their true positions. Alternative courses of future
action become correspondingly more available for cautious examination in terms of their consequences to the family and its various members. Such confronting of conflict, of course, needs to be handled very
carefully and permitted only to the extent that the total potential
resources of the family are judged to be sufficient for the experience.
Many parents can in fact cope with this challenge, given proper support and occasional individual attention from time to time to their own
maturational and relationship problems. However, sometimes the
main onus for change, through personal growth, remains with the
anorectic herself. Meanwhile, as another aspect of the individual
approach to the patient, projective art (Figure 5.3), clothes making,
and trust groups are the special responsibility of the occupational
therapist. In the picture shown, this patient, asked to paint her family,
portrayed her two brothers playing ball. Watching them, subservient
but in the same arena and allowed to pick up the ball when it dropped,
is her sister, who until recently also had anorexia nervosa. Behind the
tree, bottom right, is the childlike figure of the 24-year-old patient, ten
years an anorectic, separated off from her siblings. Above her is the
formidable figure of her mother, separated from the rest of the family
and especially from the isolated figure of the father on the left-hand
side of the picture. Although the mother dominates the patient and,
through the anorexia nervosa, retains the patient's allegiance and

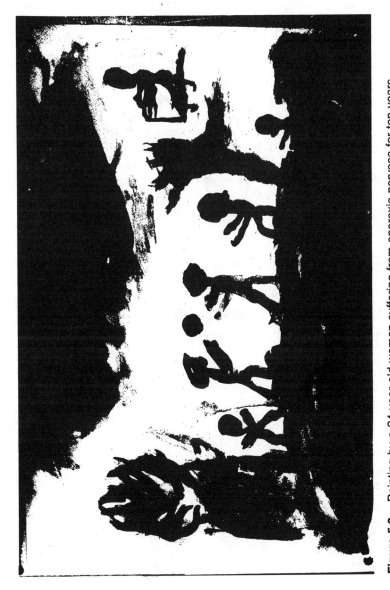

Figure 5.3. Painting by a 24-year-old woman suffering from anorexia nervosa for ten years. Reproduced with permission from Crisp, A. H. *Anorexia nervosa: Let me be.* London: Academic Press, 1980. Copyright © by Academic Press, Inc. (London) Ltd.

hence continues not to reject her, there is also a barrier between them. The patient saw this as due to their inability to share feelings and to the potential ambivalence within their relationship, which would be acutely activated once the patient had gained weight and in other ways moved away from her anorectic stance.

Progressive mobilization leads to discharge from inpatient care and continued outpatient psychotherapy over the subsequent two or so years. The initial weight gain promotes pubertal changes of the kind shown in Figures 5.4, 5.5, and 5.6. Figure 5.4 shows the maximum luteinizing hormone (LH) response, as measured by plasma level, to stimulation of the brain by a substance mirroring a natural hypothalamic agent. It can be seen that the pituitary gland was unresponsive to this stimulation so far as LH production was concerned when individuals weighed less than about 43 kg. This threshold, which must inevitably vary somewhat between individuals, probably mirrors early

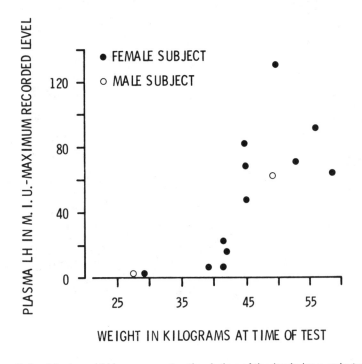

Figure 5.4.   Maximum LH response to stimulation of the brain by a substance mirroring a natural hypothalamic agent at different body weights.

Reproduced with permission from Crisp, A. H. *Anorexia nervosa: Let me be.* London: Academic Press, 1980. Copyright © by Academic Press, Inc. (London) Ltd.

features of natural puberty long before menstruation sets in. Thus, whereas on average this threshold is of the order of 41 to 44 kg, the average weight at which menstruation returns in an anorectic population is several kilograms more. Figure 5.5 shows the typical undifferentiated surge of LH that occurs as body weight approaches the 46 to 50 kg mark. This surge is more typical of early puberty than of the later, well-organized spike of high LH that appears in the blood for about 48 hours in midmenstrual cycle, heralding ovulation. Figure 5.6 shows this same surge, in this case a major one occurring in an anorectic who had been clinically and severely emaciated for over 25 years. It demonstrates that after all this time normal biological function is still possible. Despite this person's strenuous efforts and those of her would-be helpers, it can be seen that she was unable to sustain a normal weight.

It is of course important to recognize that the biological maturational changes indicated in these figures are occurring within the patient, and indeed they are usually evident in her physical status, her demeanor, and her changing behavior.

The long-term outpatient-clinic individual psychotherapy is concerned with helping the anorectic on a continuous basis to construe her

MISS A. 17yrs (Ht: 178cm)

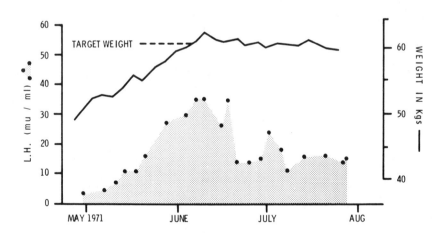

Figure 5.5. Typical undifferentiated surge of LH that occurs as body weight approaches 46 to 50 kg.

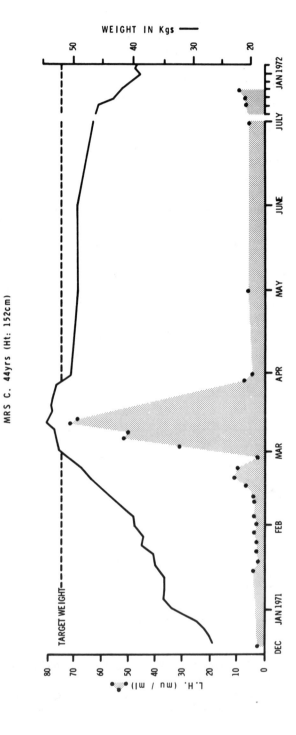

Figure 5.6. The same surge as in Figure 5.5., this a major one in a patient anorexic and emaciated for over 25 years. Reproduced with permission from Crisp, A. H. *Anorexia nervosa: Let me be.* London: Academic Press, 1980. Copyright © by Academic Press, Inc. (London) Ltd.

destiny in terms other than her body shape. In Figure 5.7 treatment aims are expressed diagrammatically for someone who fell ill at the age of 18, height 5 ft. 3 in. (160 cm), and who presented for treatment at age 21. The goals were

1. Restoration of body weight to neutral level in terms of comparability with a nonanorectic general population of similar weight and age at which the individual developed anorexia nervosa, leading to reexposure to reality of shape-related conflicts;
2. Resolution of these conflicts through development of
   (a) alternative solutions within the family, and
   (b) greater and other coping resources within the individual.

If this does not begin to happen then it is rarely that the anorectic can indefinitely sustain a mature body weight in the face of her continued panic and preoccupations.

Outcome of Treatment

What of the outcome of such treatment? There are no controlled studies. Our recent follow-up study (Hsu, Crisp, & Harding, 1979) used measures similar to those developed and used by Morgan & Russell (1975). These allow specific and general measures of both physical and psychosocial status. In trying to decide what "recovery" is, should one be aiming at ideal or normative standards? For instance, psychosexual adjustment is by no means always adequate within the general population. A previous study from this unit (Stonehill & Crisp, 1977) showed that biologically recovered anorectics were, as a group, socially phobic four years later—a more sophisticated and mature stance than that reflected in their original anorectic position and indeed one shared by quite a few "normal" people. Another recent study (Lacey, Chadbund, Crisp, Whitehead, & Stordy, 1978) has shown that "normal" adolescent females eat in a most irregular way with a highly variable calorie and carbohydrate content day by day, sometimes with consequent substantial fluctuations in body weight. For the purposes of completing the Morgan and Russell ratings we used strict criteria. For instance, for "good" outcome, weight needed to be close to general population "norms" and stable, menses present, and dietary intake stable and including adequate amounts of carbohydrate. In addition, psychosocial adjustments needed to include satisfying engagement

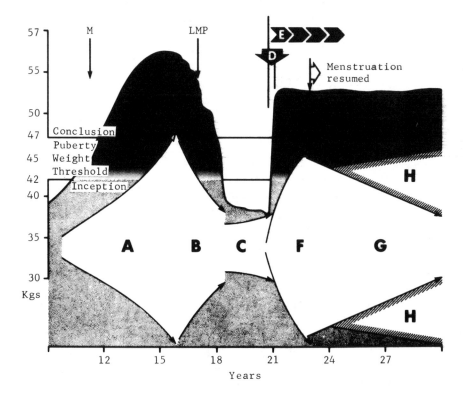

Figure 5.7. Treatment aims expressed diagrammatically. See text for explanation. Key to figure:

A. Mounting adolescent turmoil, increasingly construed in terms of body shape.
B. Resolution of this turmoil as anorexia nervosa develops.
C. Social conflict now avoided but fear of fatness persists because of constant threat of loss of control over eating and consequent weight gain. Meanwhile psychosocial maturation is impossible.
D. Body weight change during inpatient treatment.
E. Input of psychotherapy with family and patient.
F. Rekindling of adolescent conflict over shape.
G. Slowly reducing concern over shape. Increasing sense of ownership of body.
H. Growing capacity to handle adolescent problems in terms other than shape, and increasing experience of mastery over own adult destiny.

within peer relationships coupled with a reasonable capacity to cope with rejection.

Within this study Figure 5.8 shows the outcome in terms of body weight for all 100 patients, including a small proportion who did not enter treatment with us. All these patients had been severely ill with anorexia nervosa when first seen. Twenty-eight percent of the population had subsequently become involved in intensive treatment, usually for a period of about two years (see text). Body weight is an important indicator of outcome, reflecting the extent to which the avoidance posture of anorexia nervosa has been shed. Four to seven years later, 84 percent of these patients were holding a body weight above the pubertal threshold, but of these, 2 percent were obese and 18 percent were still well below average adult weight. Sixty-four percent, therefore, were sustaining a normal and stable body weight and the majority of these had regular menses.

At normal adult body weight, menstrual activity is usually rekindled although there may be considerable delay. However, these biological indices are not themselves sufficient to warrant designation of the outcome as "good." For this it is crucial for the individual to have also

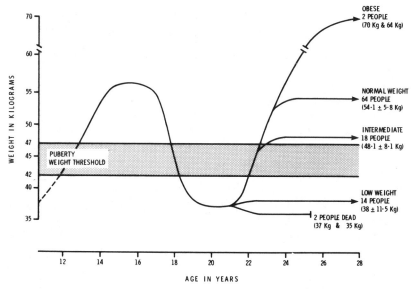

Figure 5.8. Body weight of 100 patients four to seven years after initial assessment.

consolidated an adequate psychosocial adjustment. Quite a number of these patients were still preoccupied with and sensitive about body shape, but their psychosocial adjustment was reasonable. In contrast, 14 percent remained severely ill and only 2 percent had died.

Conclusion

These figures suggest to me that such treatment as I have outlined above, aimed at altering the long-term course of the disorder for the better, is probably effective in (1) helping about 20 to 30 percent of the population to "recover" who would not otherwise have done so and (2) preventing some deaths.

References

Crisp, A. H. The possible significance of some behavioral correlates of weight and carbohydrate intake. *Journal of Psychosomatic Research,* 1967, *11,* 117–131.

Crisp, A. H. Diagnosis and outcome of anorexia nervosa: The St. George's view. *Proceedings of the Royal Society of Medicine,* 1977, *70,* 464–470.

Crisp, A. H. *Anorexia nervosa: Let me be.* London: Academic Press, 1980.

Hsu, L. K. G., Crisp, A. H., & Harding, B. Outcome of anorexia nervosa. *Lancet,* 1979, *i,* 62–65.

Lacey, J. H., Chadbund, C., Crisp, A. H., Whitehead, J., & Stordy, J. Variation in energy intake of adolescent schoolgirls. *Journal of Human Nutrition,* 1978, *32,* 419–426.

Morgan, H. G., & Russell, G. F. M. Value of family background and clinical features as predictors of long-term outcome in anorexia nervosa: Four-year follow-up study of 41 patients. *Psychological Medicine,* 1975, *5,* 353–371.

Stonehill, E., & Crisp, A. H. Psychoneurotic characteristics of patients with anorexia nervosa before and after treatment and at follow-up four to seven years later. *Journal of Psychosomatic Research,* 1977, *21,* 187–193.

6
Hypothalamic–Pituitary Function in Anorexia Nervosa and Simple Weight Loss

Robert A. Vigersky

The status of the endocrine system in disorders of weight loss, particularly anorexia nervosa, has been under intensive study for the past ten years. Impetus for the endocrinologist to investigate these patients has come from the recognition that the hypothalamus plays a central role in both the regulation of eating behavior and the control of pituitary function. Evidence for the former comes from studies in lower animals where specific lesions in the ventromedial and lateral hypothalamic nuclei produce hyperphagia and anorexia, respectively. Moreover, patients with hypothalamic tumors often present with disorders of eating behavior. The role of the hypothalamus in regulating pituitary function has been well documented. Releasing and/or inhibitory factors for all the anterior pituitary trophic hormones have been isolated and characterized in either humans or lower species. Thus, any hormonal abnormality in anorexia nervosa may be related to the eating problem by a common hypothalamic factor. This may be a specific hypothalamic "disease" or may merely be the effect of weight loss *per se* on the hypothalamus. By studying hormonal and hypothalamic function in patients with anorexia nervosa and in nonanorexic patients with weight loss (simple weight loss), these issues may be clarified.

I am indebted to D. Lynn Loriaux, M.D., for his guidance and inspiration, Arnold E. Andersen, M.D., for his excellent psychiatric assistance, Ronald Thompson, Ph.D., for performing the thermoregulatory studies, and Mrs. Barbara Kuffler for her expert secretarial assistance.

While hormonal function can be easily assessed, hunger and satiety are difficult parameters to measure in human subjects. However, the hypothalamus has several other functions that can be evaluated either directly or indirectly (Table 6.1). This chapter presents data on specific hypothalamic and pituitary functions in patients with weight loss who were studied at the National Institutes of Health (Reproduction Research Branch, National Institute of Child Health and Human Development).

All studies were performed after informed consent was obtained. Not all studies were done in each patient. Twenty-nine women were diagnosed as having anorexia nervosa (AN) by the criteria in Table 6.2

Table 6.1. Hypothalamic Functions

Thirst and water metabolism
Hunger and satiety
Temperature regulation
Endocrine regulation
Gonadotropin—LHRH
Thyrotropin—TRH
Growth hormone—Somatostatin
ACTH—CRF
Prolactin—PIF (Dopamine)

Table 6.2. Diagnostic Criteria for Anorexia Nervosa

For a diagnosis of anorexia nervosa, A through E are required.
A.   Age of onset prior to 25.
B.   Anorexia with accompanying weight loss of at least 25 percent of original body weight.
C.   A distorted, implacable attitude toward eating, food or weight that overrides hunger, admonitions, reassurance, and threats; e.g., (1) denial of illness with a failure to recognize nutritional needs; (2) apparent enjoyment in losing weight with overt manifestation that food refusal is a pleasurable indulgence; (3) a desired body image of extreme thinness with overt evidence that it is rewarding to the patient to achieve and maintain this state; and (4) unusual hoarding or handling of food.
D.   No known medical illness that could account for the anorexia and weight loss.
E.   No other known psychiatric disorder with particular reference to primary affective disorders, schizophrenia, obsessive–compulsive, and phobic neurosis.
F.   At least two of the following manifestations: (1) amenorrhea; (2) lanugo hair; (3) bradycardia (persistent resting pulse of 60 or less); (4) periods of overactivity; (5) episodes of bulimia; and (6) vomiting (may be self-induced).

From Feighner, Robin, Guze, Woodruff, Winokur, & Munoz, 1972

(Feighner, Robins, Guze, Woodruff, Winokur, & Munoz, 1972). These criteria have proved to be extremely reliable for making this diagnosis. Up to 15 years after diagnosis of AN, other psychiatric or organic disorders were not found. This is not to say that AN cannot present atypically. However, these deviations from the criteria are quantitative, not qualitative. The diagnosis of simple weight loss (SWL) (also referred to as "anorexoid") was made in 19 women who presented with secondary amenorrhea, which developed while they were losing moderate amounts of weight. This weight loss was deemed appropriate by physicians, peers, and family and these women had normal ideation about food and body image without a "relentless pursuit of thinness." No patient, in up to ten years of follow-up, moved from the SWL to the AN group. Table 6.3 shows the age, weight, and percent below ideal body weight (based on the Metropolitan Life Insurance tables) of these two groups. It should be noted that the anorexia nervosa group is somewhat older than the average anorexia nervosa patient. This is likely to be due to the fact that NIH represents a tertiary (or quaternary) referral center for anorexia nervosa patients. The SWL patients had only moderate amounts of weight loss compared to the anorexia nervosa group. These two patients' groups were compared to 20 normal women in the early follicular phase of their menstrual cycle.

Table 6.3. Clinical Data on Patients with Weight Loss

	Age	Weight	% Below IBW
Anorexia nervosa	24 ± 8.4*	34.3 ± 6.6	32 ± 10
Simple weight loss	23 ± 5.7	44.8 ± 7.6	15 ± 10

*mean ± S.D.

Pituitary-End Organ Function (Table 6.4)

Growth Hormone

Basal serum growth hormone (GH) levels were significantly higher in AN compared to controls ($p < 0.001$) and to SWL ($p < 0.05$). The SWL patients also had significantly higher serum GH levels than controls ($p < 0.05$). The level of GH was directly correlated with the percent below ideal body weight (IBW) in the AN group ($r=0.60$; $p<0.005$) (Vigersky, Loriaux, Andersen, & Lipsett, 1976a). The response

⊙

Table 6.4. Pituitary-End Organ Function in Normal Women and in Patients with Anorexia Nervosa or Simple Weight Loss

Hormone	Normal Women	Simple Weight Loss (SWL)	Anorexia Nervosa (AN)
Growth hormone (ng/dl)	2.3 ± 1.0‡	23.1 ± 2.4*†	48.1 ± 11.2**
Prolactin (ng/dl)	16.2 ± 1.2	20.0 ± 1.2	19.4 ± 3.1
TSH (μU/ml)	ND in 77%§	ND in 25%	ND in 30%
	7.6 in 23%	4.6 in 75%	6.0 in 70%
Free thyroxine (ng/dl)	1.5 ± 0.05	1.3 ± 0.14	1.5 ± 0.04
Triiodothyronine (ng/dl)	156 ± 4.4	117 ± 17.1‖	78 ± 24*
Cortisol (μg/dl)	14.4 ± 1.0	12.6 ± 1.7	14.8 ± 1.3
LH (mIU/ml)	7.9 ± 2.6	8.3 ± 2.3	3.9 ± 0.5**
FSH (mIU/ml)	15.3 ± 1.0	9.4 ± 1.2†‖	5.6 ± 1.1*

* $p<0.01$ AN or SWL vs. normal
** $p<0.001$ AN or SWL vs. normal
† $p<0.05$ AN or SWL vs. normal
‖ $p<0.05$ AN vs. SWL
§ ND denotes not detectable
‡ values are mean ± SE

to provocative stimuli was normal (data not shown), though others have found blunted GH responses to insulin-induced hypoglycemia in both AN and SWL (Brauman & Gregoire, 1975; Devlin, 1975; Hirvonen, Seppala, Karonen, & Adlercreutz, 1977). Furthermore, paradoxical increases in GH after glucose loading (Alvarez, Dimas, Castro, Rossman, Vanderlaan, & Vanderlaan, 1972; Casper, Davis, & Panday, 1977), TRH-induced GH release (Casper et al., 1977), and the failure of GH to respond to apomorphine (Macaron, Wilbur, Green, & Freinkel, 1978) have been found by others. These results suggest that while the GH secretory ability of the pituitary is normal, hypothalamic regulation of GH is abnormal. The reason for the elevated GH levels is not clear. It may signify an attempt to defend against the hypoglycemia often seen in AN. At the very least, the fact that GH is elevated differentiates the AN patient from someone with hypopituitarism.

Prolactin

Patients with AN and SWL have normal basal serum prolactin with a quantitatively normal response to TRH (Figure 6.1). Similar results have been found by others (Macaron et al., 1978; Wakeling, DeSouza, Gore, Sabur, Kingstone, & Boss, 1979).

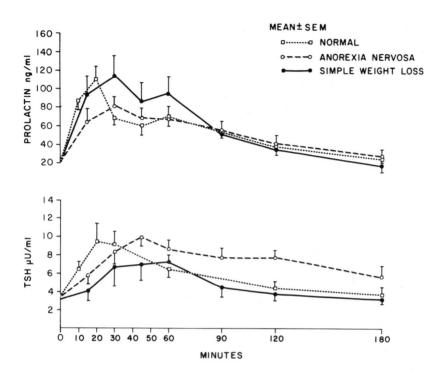

Figure 6.1. Response of prolactin (upper panel) and thyrotropin (TSH) (lower panel) to 500 μg of TRH i.v. given at time 0 in normal women, anorexia nervosa patients, and patients with simple weight loss.

Thyrotropin and Thyroid Hormones

Basal serum thyrotropin (TSH) and the quantitative response to thyrotropin releasing hormone (TRH) are normal in both AN and SWL (Figure 6.1). However, there are changes in the levels of peripheral thyroid hormones that have led to some confusion. Total serum thyroxine (T4) levels are either low or low normal, though "free" T4 is normal. In addition, serum T3 levels are significantly lower in AN than in both normals ($p<0.01$) and SWL ($p<0.05$), and reverse T3 (3,3',5'-triiodothyronine) levels are elevated (Burman, Vigersky, Loriaux, Strum, Djuh, Wright, & Wartofsky, 1977). The clinical observations of bradycardia, dry skin, constipation, and hypothermia and the laboratory studies showing low basal metabolic rate, prolonged achilles reflex time, hypercarotenemia, and hypothyroid-like alterations in testosterone metabolism (Bradlow, Boyar, O'Connor, Zumoff, & Hellman, 1976; Frumar, Meldrum, & Judd, 1979; Hurd, Palumbo, & Gharib, 1977) in conjunction with the above-noted peripheral thyroid hormone levels and TRH responses, suggest that anorexia nervosa patients are centrally euthyroid while peripherally hypothyroid. However, treatment with thyroid hormone is *not* indicated since it appears that these peripheral changes are adaptive to the decreased caloric intake.

Corticotropin and Cortisol

Basal serum cortisol levels are normal in both AN and SWL, though there are abnormalities of the circadian rhythm (*vide infra*). These patients respond normally to insulin-induced hypoglycemia or metopirone with increases in serum cortisol and/or urinary 17-hydroxycorticosteroids (Hirvonen et al., 1977; Marks & Bannister, 1963; Vigersky, Andersen, Thompson, & Loriaux, 1977). Others have measured the daily production rate of cortisol in AN and found it to be either normal or elevated (Boyar, Hellman, Roffwarg, Katz, Zumoff, O'Connor, Bradlow, & Fukushima, 1977; Walsh, Katz, Levin, Kream, Fukushima, Hellman, Weiner, & Zumoff, 1978). The elevation of cortisol production, like that of GH, may be a counterregulatory response to the hypoglycemia produced by insulin hypersensitivity of AN (Mecklenburg, Loriaux, Thompson, Andersen, & Lipsett, 1974). This insulin hypersensitivity may be mediated via an increased number of insulin receptors (Wachslicht-Rodbard, Gross, Rodbard, Ebert, & Roth, 1979). Another interpretation of the elevated cortisol secretion may be that it is related to the degree of depression and/or stress that AN patients have.

Gonodotropins and Estrogen

Serum estradiol levels in AN are usually unmeasurable (<10 pg/ml), while those in SWL, if measurable, are low to low normal. The reason for the low serum estradiol concentration is the low serum luteinizing hormone (LH) levels found in patients with AN. In fact, both basal LH and follicle stimulating hormone (FSH) are significantly lower than normal in AN ($p<0.001$ and $p<0.01$ respectively). The serum LH concentration is also lower in SWL. The normal response of LH and FSH to the exogenous administration of the hypothalamic releasing factor LHRH (LH releasing hormone) implies that the pituitary is

capable of secreting gonadotropin if only given the appropriate stimulus (Figure 6.2). Thus, the amenorrhea of both AN and SWL can be
classified as "hypothalamic." Other proof that the pituitary and ovaries
are intrinsically normal is found in the observations that chronic
LHRH administration (via pulsatile i.v. or i.m. administration) restores
LH responsiveness to LHRH to a normal adult pattern (i.e., the LH
response is greater than FSH response) and induces ovulation (Mar-

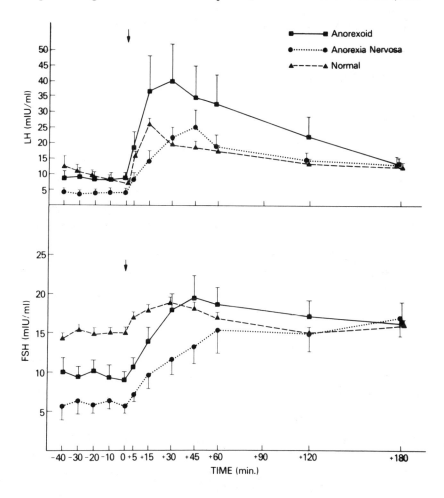

Figure 6.2.   The response of LH (upper panel) and FSH (lower panel) to 10 μg
LHRH i.v. (arrow) in normal women in the early follicular phase of
their menstrual cycle, anorexia nervosa, and simple weight loss
(anorexoid). Symbols and bars represent the mean ± S.E.

shall & Kelch, 1979; Nillius, Fries, & Wide, 1975; Yoshimoto, Moridera, & Imura, 1975). The quantitative response of LH and FSH for the entire AN and SWL group is normal. However, there is wide variation within the group with some individuals being frankly low. Subnormal LHRH responses have been found by others (Sherman, Halmi, & Zamudio, 1975). There is a significant correlation between the quantitative response of LH and FSH in AN and the severity of weight loss ($p<0.05$). In addition, others have shown that with nutritional rehabilitation, the response of LH to LHRH improves.

Hypothalamic Function (Table 6.5)

The discovery and development for clinical use of the hypothalamic releasing factors, particularly TRH and LHRH, has permitted the endocrinologist to dissect out the precise level at which an hormonal deficiency or excess occurs. This is seen most clearly with the assessment of gonadal status in AN and SWL, where the ultimate level of deficiency is the hypothalamus. In addition, techniques have been developed that allow the direct and indirect assessment of certain hypothalamic functions. Thus, it is possible to estimate hypothalamic function in a particular patient by combining the assessment of hormonal status with tests of specific hypothalamic function. The principles upon which the diagnosis of hypothalamic dysfunction can be made are shown in Table 6.6.

Thermoregulation

Patients with AN often complain of feeling cold, and measurement of their body temperature may reveal basal hypothermia in many cases. How these patients and those with SWL respond to thermal stress has been assessed in an environmental chamber. Subjects are placed in the chamber for 30 to 60 minutes clad in bathing suits, with a rectal thermistor in place. They are tested on different days at environmental temperatures of 49°C (12 percent relative humidity) and 10°C. The response of normal individuals to these temperatures is an initial paradoxical rise in the cold (due to peripheral vasodilatation, which shunts warm blood to the core) and an initial paradoxical decrease in the heat (due to peripheral vasodilatation which shunts blood away from the core). However, by the end of the test period, the core

Table 6.5. Hypothalamic Function in Patients with Anorexia Nervosa and Simple Weight Loss

	Percent with Abnormal Tests	
	AN	SWL
Thermoregulation		
Heat	86*	100
Cold	85*	91
Partial diabetes insipidus	44	27
Time of pituitary hormone response		
after TRH		
TSH	80*	75
Prolactin	29	16
after LHRH		
LH	93	74*
FSH	76	26*
Diurnal variation of cortisol	54	20

*Severity of abnormality correlated with percent below IBW

Table 6.6. Diagnosis of Hypothalamic Dysfunction

1. No abnormality of end organ function not attributable to a pituitary cause.
2. No abnormality of pituitary function not attributable to a suprasellar cause.
3. An abnormality of a specific hypothalamic function.

temperature has returned to within 0.5°C of the starting temperature and has plateaued. The function $\Delta T°/\Delta t$, that is, the rate of change of temperature at the end of the test period, is near 0. Patients with SWL and AN have several abnormalities of thermoregulation. As shown in Figure 6.3, the $\Delta T°/\Delta t$ in both groups are significantly different from normal women in both the heat and cold. The SWL group is intermediate in severity between AN and normal in the heat while equal to AN in the cold. Not only do most of the AN patients have absence of the paradoxical changes in both the heat and cold, but the severity of their thermoregulatory abnormality is significantly correlated with the percent below IBW (Figure 6.4). In addition, shivering, another hypothalamic function, was not present in any of the AN patients. Thermoregulation remained abnormal in two patients studied after weight gain. In these patients, one cannot distinguish between the possibilities that

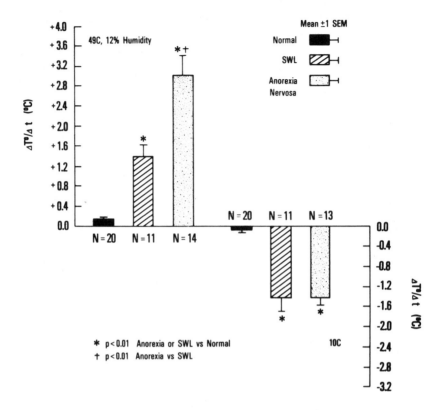

Figure 6.3. Mean ± S.E. rate of change of core temperature per hour ($\Delta T°/\Delta t$) in the heat (left panel) and cold (right panel) in normal women, anorexia nervosa, and simple weight loss (SWL). Temperature was recorded at one-minute intervals via a rectal thermistor.

weight loss induced permanent hypothalamic damage or that the hypothalamic dysfunction of AN is unrelated to the previous weight loss.

Water Conservation

Antidiuretic hormone (ADH) is produced by the supraoptic and para-ventricular nuclei of the hypothalamus, though released from the posterior pituitary. Most disorders of pituitary ADH secretion are a result of abnormal hypothalamic ADH synthesis. The complete deficiency of ADH produces the syndrome of diabetes insipidus, while

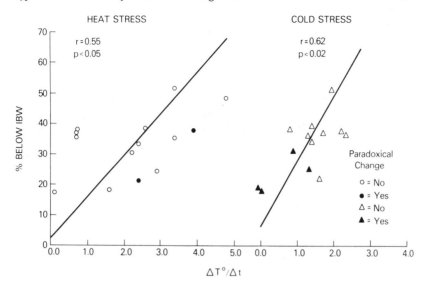

Figure 6.4.   Linear regression analyses of the severity of weight loss (percent below IBW) in patients with anorexia nervosa vs. the rate of change of core temperature per hour ($\Delta T°/\Delta t$) in the heat (49°C, 12 percent relative humidity) and cold (10°C). Paradoxical change refers to the initial rise in the cold or fall in the heat seen in normal subjects.

less severe abnormalities produce "partial" diabetes insipidus, a disorder that is usually not clinically apparent. In the absence of the general availability of direct measurement of ADH, the diagnosis of complete or "partial" diabetes insipidus can be made using the overnight dehydration test. After 12 or more hours of fasting, normal individuals will maximally concentrate their urine due to the elaboration of endogenous ADH. The administration of exogenous ADH (5 units of aqueous pitressin) will not cause a further increase in urine osmolarity. In contrast, patients with complete diabetes insipidus do not increase their urine osmolarity after water deprivation and respond to the administration of exogenous vasopressin with a dramatic rise in urine osmolarity. Patients with "partial" diabetes insipidus concentrate their urine submaximally, yet respond to exogenous pitressin with a further (greater than 10 percent) rise in urine osmolarity.

When patients with AN and SWL are tested with a water-deprivation test for the presence of "partial" diabetes insipidus, 44 percent of the former and 27 percent of the latter are found to have this disorder (see Table 6.5).

*Qualitative Response of Pituitary
Hormones to Hypothalamic
Releasing Factors*

Delayed or prolonged release of TSH after TRH injection has been found in patients with organic diseases of the hypothalamus but not in patients with pituitary disorders (Faglia, Beck-Peccoz, Ferrari, Ambrosi, Spada, Travaglini, & Paracchi, 1975; Hall, Ornston, Besser, Cryer, & McKendrik, 1972). Thus, abnormal kinetics in conjunction with a normal quantitative response to the releasing factor implies hypothalamic dysfunction. This can also be extended to observations of the kinetics of LH and FSH responses. For example, as seen in Figure 6.5, most normal women respond with a peak of LH after LHRH at 15 minutes, while most women with AN have significantly later peak hormone levels. SWL patients are intermediate. There is also a delay in peak FSH levels after LHRH and in peak prolactin and TSH after TRH in AN and SWL (Figure 6.6). Similar delay in TSH peaks have been shown by others in AN (Aro, Lamberg, & Pelkonen, 1977) and in protein–calorie malnutrition (Pimstone, Becker, & Hendricks, 1973). The time of the peak LH and FSH levels after LHRH were

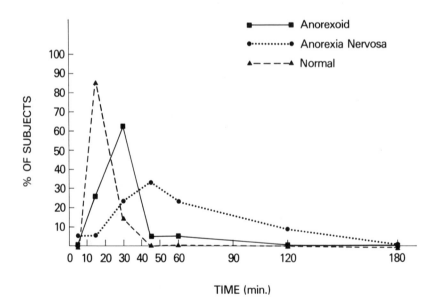

Figure 6.5.   The distribution of the time of peak LH levels after 10 μg of LHRH in normal women (*N* = 7), anorexia nervosa patients (*N* = 21), and simple weight loss [anorexoid patients (*N* = 19)].

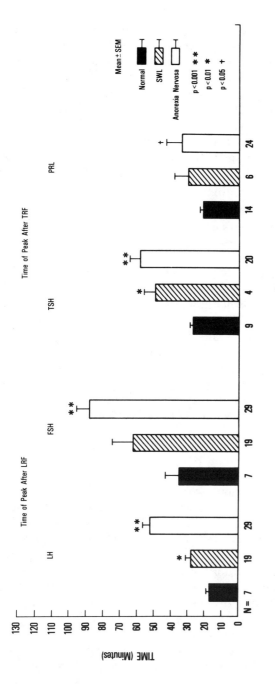

Figure 6.6. Time of peak serum LH and FSH levels after 10 μg of LHRH (LRF) and of peak TSH and prolactin after 500 μg of TRH (TRF) in normal women, anorexia nervosa, and simple weight loss (SWL).

significantly correlated with the severity of weight loss in the SWL group ($p<0.05$ and <0.01, respectively). The lateness of the TSH peak after TRH was significantly correlated with the severity of weight loss in AN ($p<0.01$).

The functional significance of delayed hormone secretion is unclear. The severity of the delay is not correlated with the basal or releasing- factor stimulatable levels of LH, FSH, TRH, or prolactin. It may be such a qualitative, rather than a quantitative, difference in trophic hormone response that explains the failure of women with AN or SWL to have regular menstrual cycles (Vigersky, Loriaux, Andersen, Mecklenburg, & Vaitukaitis, 1976b).

Other Indirect Parameters of Hypothalamic Function

Diurnal variation of cortisol is controlled through hypothalamic mechanisms. Patients with AN (54 percent) and SWL (20 percent) have failure to decrease afternoon plasma cortisol levels to less than half of their morning levels. This has been confirmed by others (Aro, Lamberg, & Pelkonen, 1977; Frankel, & Jenkins, 1975), though disputed by Boyar and associates (1977), who attribute the failure of afternoon cortisols to decrease to a prolonged cortisol half-life.

As noted above, the response of GH to provocative and suppressive stimuli in AN indicates that they have abnormal hypothalamic regulation. These studies have not been performed in SWL patients.

Discussion

The findings in our patients with AN and SWL and those of others in similar groups suggest that there is marked dysfunction of the hypothalamus. The pituitary is basically normal, with any abnormality attributable to a hypothalamic factor. Similarly, end-organ function is also basically normal. In addition to the fact that there is hypothalamic dysfunction, what is striking is that most of the abnormalities at all levels are related to the weight loss. Thus, within the AN or SWL group there are correlations of the severity of the abnormality and the amount of weight loss. Furthermore, in general the SWL group has abnormalities that are intermediate in severity relative to those in AN. These data argue strongly that there is no specific hypothalamic disease in AN, but rather the hypothalamic changes are secondary to the weight loss *per se*.

The mechanism by which weight loss causes the hypothalamic dysfunction found in AN and SWL is unclear. With respect to gonadotropin secretion, it has been proposed that a critical amount of fatness is necessary for menstrual function (Frisch, 1977; Frisch & McArthur, 1974). The hypogonadotropic hypogonadism associated with decreased fatness may be mediated via metabolic activities that occur in the fat itself. Fat actively metabolizes testosterone and androstenedione to estradiol and estrone, respectively, and such changes in the peripheral metabolism of the sex steroids may modulate the secretion of gonadotropins (Nimrod & Ryan, 1975; Schindler, Ebert, & Friedrich, 1972).

Other factors undoubtedly come into play in AN patients. For example, the weight loss hypothesis does not explain the finding that 71 percent of AN patients become amenorrheic before or coinciding with weight loss (Fries, 1977) and 50 percent fail to resume menstruation after weight is regained (Bell, Harkness, Loraine, & Russell, 1966; Russell, 1972). Among these other factors, stress and exercise (or activity) are likely to be contributory (Fries, Nillius, & Pettersson, 1974). Stress-induced amenorrhea is a poorly defined yet frequently used diagnosis. No endocrine studies of a "pure" stress-induced amenorrhea group have been performed. Undoubtedly such patients are included in those patients studied with "hypothalamic" amenorrhea in whom hypogonadotropic hypogonadism has been found (Lachelin & Yen, 1978; Rakoff, Rigg, & Yen, 1978; Yen, Rebar, Vandenburg, & Judd, 1973). Similarly, exercise-induced amenorrhea in long-distance runners and ballet dancers has been found to be hypogonadotropic (Erdelyi, 1976; Feicht, Johnson, Martin, Sparkes, & Wagner, 1978; McArthur, Bullen, Beitins, Pagano, Badger, & Klibanski, 1980; Warren, 1980). In a fascinating study of the interrelationship of weight and exercise (and perhaps stress) to menstrual function, Warren has found that menses resumes in ballet dancers who are at or below their critical body fatness when they stop practicing for reasons of injury or vacation (Warren, 1980). This occurs without an increase in body weight or fatness. She proposes that ballet practice imposes an "energy drain," which prevents menses. AN patients are generally hyperactive and undoubtedly under a great deal of stress. Thus, the amenorrhea caused by hypogonadotropic hypogonadism is most likely to be multifactoral in origin, some or all of which is mediated via suprahypothalamic factors.

Though the thermoregulatory changes seem to be clearly related to weight loss, the mechanism may be mediated via changes in carbohydrate metabolism. Hypothermia is found in hypoglycemic patients and may be mediated via intracerebral glucopenia. There is a 56 percent incidence of hypoglycemia in AN and a significant correlation between basal body temperature and fasting blood sugar ($p < 0.05$) (Vigersky, 1977).

Conclusion

It would be fair to say that while its mechanism remains a mystery, weight loss in both psychologically normal and abnormal individuals induces numerous changes in endocrine status and hypothalamic function. Some aspects of these changes are clinically apparent (e.g., amenorrhea), others silent (e.g., partial diabetes insipidus), while still others are more apparent than real (e.g., abnormalities in thyroid hormone tests). With the information about the effects of weight loss on the endocrine system in mind, the physician should be able to correctly interpret the sometimes confusing data obtained in AN patients.

References

Alvarez, L. C., Dimas, C. O., Castro, A., Rossman, L. G., Vanderlaan, E. F., & Vanderlaan, W. P. Growth hormone in malnutrition. *Journal of Clinical Endocrinology and Metabolism*, 1972, *34*, 400–409.

Aro, A., Lamberg, B. A., & Pelkonen, R. Hypothalamic endocrine dysfunction in anorexia nervosa. *Acta Endocrinologica*, 1977, *85*, 673–683.

Bell, E. T., Harkness, R. A., Loraine, J. A., & Russell, G. F. M. Hormone assay studies in patients with anorexia nervosa. *Acta Endocrinologica*, 1966, *51*, 140–148.

Boyar, R. M., Hellman, L. D., Roffwarg, H. P., Katz, J., Zumoff, B., O'Connor, J., Bradlow, H. L., & Fukushima, D. K. Cortisol secretion and metabolism in anorexia nervosa. *New England Journal of Medicine*, 1977, *296*, 190–193.

Bradlow, H. L., Boyar, R. M., O'Connor, J., Zumoff, B., & Hellman, L. Hypothyroid-like alterations in testosterone metabolism in anorexia nervosa. *Journal of Clinical Endocrinology and Metabolism*, 1976, *43*, 571–574.

Brauman, H., & Gregoire, F. The growth hormone response to insulin hypoglycemia in anorexia nervosa and control underweight or normal subjects. *European Journal of Clinical Investigation*, 1975, *5*, 289–295.

Bruch, H. *Eating disorders: Obesity, anorexia nervosa and the person within.* New York: Basic Books, 1973.

Burman, K. D., Vigersky, R. A., Loriaux, D. L., Strum, D., Djuh, Y., Wright, F. D., Wartofsky, L. Investigations concerning thyroxine deiodinative pathways in patients with anorexia nervosa. In R. A. Vigersky (Ed.)., *Anorexia nervosa.* New York: Raven Press, 1977, pp. 255–261.

Casper, R. G., Davis, J. M., & Panday, G. N. The effect of the nutritional status and weight changes on hypothalamic function tests in anorexia nervosa. In R. A. Vigersky (Ed.), *Anorexia nervosa.* New York: Raven Press, 1977, pp. 137–147.

Devlin, J. G. Obesity and anorexia nervosa: A study of growth hormone release. *Journal of the Irish Medical Association,* 1975, *68,* 227–231.

Erdelyi, G. J. Effects of exercise on the menstrual cycle. *Physician and Sports Medicine,* 1976, *4,* 79–81.

Faglia, G. P., Beck-Peccoz, P., Ferrari, C., Ambrosi, B., Spada, A., Travaglini, P., & Paracchi, S. Plasma thyrotropin- releasing hormone in patients with pituitary and hypothalamic disorders. *Journal of Clinical Endocrinology and Metabolism,* 1975, *37,* 596–601.

Feicht, C. B., Johnson, T. S., Martin, B. J., Sparkes, K. E., & Wagner, W. W., Jr. Secondary amenorrhea in athletes. *Lancet,* 1978, *2,* 1145–1146.

Feighner, J. P., Robins, E., Guze, S. B., Woodruff, R. A., Jr., Winokur, G., & Munoz, R. Diagnostic criteria for use in psychiatric research. *Archives of General Psychiatry,* 1972, *26,* 57–63.

Frankel, R. J., & Jenkins, J. S. Hypothalamic-pituitary function in anorexia nervosa. *Acta Endocrinologica,* 1975, *78,* 209–221.

Fries, H. Studies on secondary amenorrhea, anorectic behavior, and body-image perception: Importance for the early recognition of anorexia nervosa. In R. A. Vigersky (Ed.), *Anorexia nervosa.* New York: Raven Press, 1977, pp. 163–176.

Fries, H., Nillius, S. J., & Pettersson, F. Epidemiology of secondary amenorrhea. II. A retrospective evaluation of etiology with special regard to psychogenic factor and weight loss. *American Journal of Obstetrics and Gynecology,* 1974, *118,* 473–479.

Frisch, R. E. Food intake, fatness, and reproductive ability. In R. A. Vigersky (Ed.), *Anorexia nervosa.* New York: Raven Press, 1977, pp. 149–161.

Frisch, R. E., & McArthur, J. W. Menstrual cycles: Fatness as a determinant of minimum weight for height necessary for their maintenance or onset. *Science,* 1974, *185,* 949–951.

Frumar, A. M., Meldrum, D. R., & Judd, H. L. Hypercarotenemia in hypothalamic amenorrhea. *Fertility and Sterility,* 1979, *32,* 261–264.

Hall, R., Ornston, B. J., Besser, G. M., Cryer, R. J., & McKendrick, M. The thyrotropin-releasing hormone test in disease of the pituitary and hypothalamus. *Lancet,* 1972, *1,* 759–763.

Hirvonen, E., Seppala, M., Karonen, S. L., & Adlercreutz, H. Luteinizing hormone responses to luteinizing hormone releasing hormone and growth hormone and cortisol responses to insulin induced hypoglycemia in functional secondary amenorrhea. *Acta Endocrinologica,* 1977, *84,* 225–236.

Hurd, H. P., II, Palumbo, P. J., & Gharib, H. Hypothalamic-endocrine dysfunction in anorexia nervosa. *Mayo Clinic Proceedings,* 1977, *52,* 711–716.

Lachelin, G. C. L., & Yen, S. S. C. Hypothalamic chronic anovulation. *American Journal of Obstetrics and Gynecology*, 1978, *130*, 825–831.

Macaron, C., Wilbur, J. F., Green, O., & Freinkel, N. Studies of growth hormone (GH), thyrotropin (TSH) and prolactin (PRL) secretion in anorexia nervosa. *Psychoneuroendocrinology*, 1978, *3*, 181–185.

Marks, V., & Bannister, R. G. Pituitary and adrenal function in undernutrition with mental illness (including anorexia nervosa). *British Journal of Psychiatry*, 1963, *109*, 480–484.

Marshall, J. F., & Kelch, R. P. Low dose pulsatile gonadotropin-releasing hormone in anorexia nervosa: A model of human pubertal development. *Journal of Clinical Endocrinology and Metabolism*, 1979, *49*, 712–718.

McArthur, J. W., Bullen, B. A., Beitins, I. Z., Pagano, M., Badger, T. M., Klibanski, A. Hypothalamic amenorrhea in runners of normal body composition. *Endocrine Research Communications*, 1980, *7*, 13–25.

Mecklenburg, R. S., Loriaux, D. L., Thompson, R. H., Andersen, A. E., & Lipsett, M. B. Hypothalamic dysfunction in patients with anorexia nervosa. *Medicine*, 1974, *53*, 147–159.

Nillius, S. J., Fries, H., & Wide, L. Successful induction of follicular maturation and ovulation by prolonged treatment with LH-releasing hormone in women with anorexia nervosa. *American Journal of Obstetrics and Gynecology*, 1975, *122*, 921–928.

Nimrod, A., & Ryan, K. J. Aromatization of androgens by human abdominal and breast fat tissue. *Journal of Clinical Endocrinology and Metabolism*, 1975, *40*, 367–372.

Pimstone, B., Becker, D., & Hendricks, S. TSH response to synthetic thyrotropin-releasing hormone in protein-calorie malnutrition. *Journal of Clinical Endocrinology and Metabolism*, 1973, *39*, 779–783.

Rakoff, J. S., Rigg, L. A., & Yen, S. S. C. The impairment of progesterone-induced pituitary release of prolactin and gonadotropin in patients with hypothalamic chronic anovulation. *American Journal of Obstetrics and Gynecology*, 1978, *130*, 807–812.

Russell, G. F. M. Psychological and nutritional factors in disturbance of menstrual function and ovulation. *Postgraduate Medical Journal*, 1972, *48*, 10–13.

Schindler, A. E., Ebert, A., & Friedrich, E. Conversion of androstenedione to estrone by human fat tissue. *Journal of Clinical Endocrinology and Metabolism*, 1972, *35*, 627–630.

Sherman, B. M., Halmi, K. A., & Zamudio, R. LH and FSH response to gonadotropin-releasing hormone in anorexia nervosa: Effect of nutritional rehabilitation. *Journal of Clinical Endocrinology and Metabolism*, 1975, *41*, 135–142.

Vigersky, R. A. (Ed.). *Anorexia nervosa*. New York: Raven Press, 1977.

Vigersky, R. A., Andersen, A. E., Thompson, R. H., & Loriaux, D. L. Hypothalamic dysfunction in secondary amenorrhea associated with simple weight loss. *New England Journal of Medicine*, 1977, *297*, 1141–1145.

Vigersky, R. A., Loriaux, D. L., Andersen, A. E., & Lipsett, M. B. Anorexia nervosa: Behavioral and hypothalamic aspects. *Journal of Clinical Endocrinology and Metabolism*, 1976, *5*, 517–535.(a)

Vigersky, R. A., Loriaux, D. L., Andersen, A. E., Mecklenburg, R. S., & Vaitukaitis, J. L. Delayed pituitary hormone response to LRF and TRF in patients with anorexia nervosa and with secondary amenorrhea associated with simple weight loss. *Journal of Clinical Endocrinology and Metabolism*, 1976, *43*, 893–900. (b)

Wachslicht-Rodbard, H., Gross, H. A., Rodbard, D., Ebert, M. H., & Roth, J. Increased insulin binding to erythrocytes in anorexia nervosa. *New England Journal of Medicine*, 1979, *300*, 882–887.

Wakeling, A., DeSouza, V. F. A., Gore, M. B. R., Sabur, M., Kingstone, D., & Boss, A. M. Amenorrhea, body weight and serum hormone concentrations, with particular reference to prolactin and thyroid hormones in anorexia nervosa. *Psychological Medicine*, 1979, *9*, 265–272.

Walsh, B. T., Katz, J. L., Levin, J., Kream, J., Fukushima, D. K., Hellman, L. D., Weiner, H., & Zumoff, B. Adrenal activity in anorexia nervosa. *Psychosomatic Medicine*, 1978, *40*, 499–506.

Warren, M. P. The effects of exercise on pubertal progression and reproductive function in girls. *Journal of Clinical Endocrinology and Metabolism*, 1980, *51*, 1150–1157.

Yen, S. S. C., Rebar, R., Vandenburg, G., & Judd, H. Hypothalamic amenorrhea and hypogonadotropinism: Responses to synthetic LRF. *Journal of Clinical Endocrinology and Metabolism*, 1973, *36*, 811–816.

Yoshimoto, T., Moridera, K., & Imura, H. Restoration of normal pituitary gonadotropin reserve by administration of luteinizing-hormone-releasing hormone in patients with hypogonadotropic hypogonadism. *New England Journal of Medicine*, 1975, *292*, 242–245.

7

Reproductive Hormone Profiles in Male Anorexia Nervosa before during, and after Restoration of Body Weight to Normal: A Study of Twelve Patients

Arthur H. Crisp   L. K. G. Hsu

C. N. Chen   M. Wheeler

With improved diagnostic criteria and more refined measurements of various hormonal levels, renewed interest in the endocrine aspects of anorexia nervosa has produced a deluge of publications (Isaacs, 1979). Most of the data, however, have been derived from investigations of female patients and little is known about the reproductive hormone profile in the male anorectic.

Method and Subjects

Between 1974 and 1979, 12 male patients diagnosed as suffering from anorexia nervosa were admitted for treatment to Atkinson Morley's Hospital, London, under the care of one of us (AHC). The diagnostic criteria of the syndrome in the male are outlined in Table 7.1.

Table 7.1   Diagnostic Criteria for Anorexia Nervosa in the Male

---

1. Weight loss of > 25 percent premorbid weight.
2. Implacable mental attitude of "weight phobia."
3. Behavior directed toward weight loss such as food refusal, vomiting, purgative abuse, and excessive exercising.
4. Loss of sexual interest/potency.
5. Age of onset before 25.

We have investigated plasma testosterone levels on admission and thereafter during treatment involving full restoration of body weight and psychotherapy (Crisp, 1967) in ten of these patients, while plasma luteinizing hormone (LH) levels have been similarly studied in eight and follicle stimulating hormone (FSH) in six subjects. Finally, in five subjects the pituitary response to 50 μg LH/RH has been investigated, four on two occasions and one on three occasions. In all five subjects the first test was performed when they were at a low weight soon after their admission. In two subjects the test was repeated at around 85 percent matched population mean weight (MPMW), and in four subjects at "target" weight (MPMW at age of onset of illness). Only one of the patients had any medication during his refeeding treatment.

Results

Individual Hormones

Testosterone.   Plasma testosterone levels have been found to increase with weight gain. Using analysis of covariance, plasma testosterone in the ten subjects is significantly correlated with body weight expressed as a percentage of matched population mean weight (MPMW), with a regression coefficient of 0.105 (F = 48.03, df = 8, $p < 0.001$). However, the testosterone levels at target weight are still often below normal levels (normal range 10–30 nmol/L) (Figure 7.1).

Luteinizing Hormone.   Plasma LH levels in the eight subjects are also significantly correlated with body weight expressed as a percentage of MPMW. Analysis of covariance, F = 11.11, df = 6, $p < 0.001$, yields regression coefficient 0.041 (Figure 7.2).

Follicular Stimulating Hormone.   This is not correlated with body weight expressed as a percentage of MPMW.

LH/RH Study.   The LH response seemed to be related not so

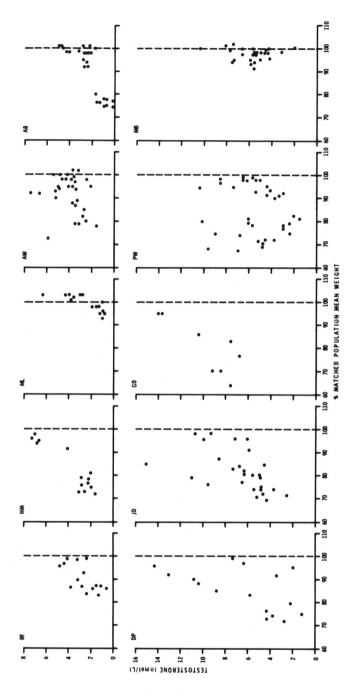

Figure 7.1. Plasma testosterone levels in ten males with anorexia nervosa studied during the time that they gained weight to normal (matched population mean weight) levels. (Normal range 10–30 nmol/L)

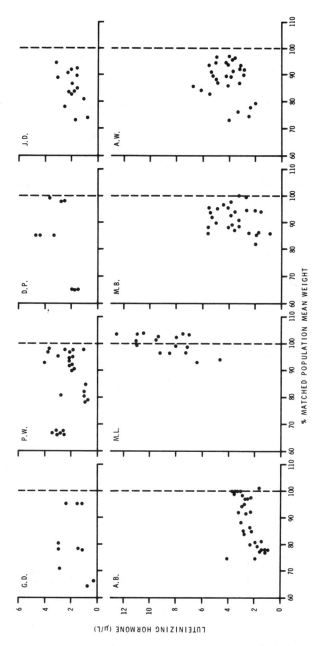

Figure 7.2. Plasma luteinizing hormone levels in eight males with anorexia nervosa studied during the time that they gained weight to normal (matched population mean weight) levels.

much to percentage MPMW but to the actual weight of the subject, irrespective of height.

1. At low weight, two subjects with a weight of 27 kg and 37.6 kg, respectively, showed little or no RH response (Figures 7.3 and 7.4). Another two, whose weights were low in terms of their percentage MPMW (70 percent and 75 percent respectively), but which were around 46 ± 2 kg, instead showed an enhanced LH response with delayed peak (Figures 7.5 and 7.6).
2. Two subjects tested at around 85 percent MPMW also showed a dissimilar response. One whose weight was 44 kg had an enhanced LH response (Figure 7.3) while the other whose

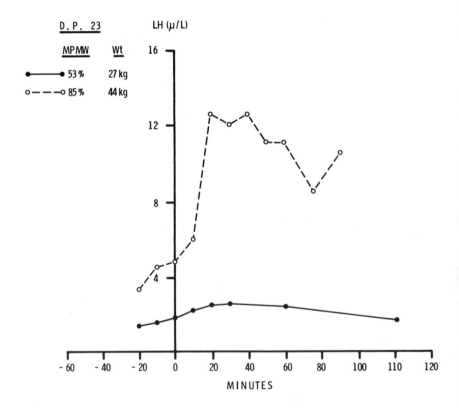

Figure 7.3. LH responses to 50 μg LHRH in males with anorexia nervosa studied during the time that they gained weight to normal (matched population mean weight) levels.

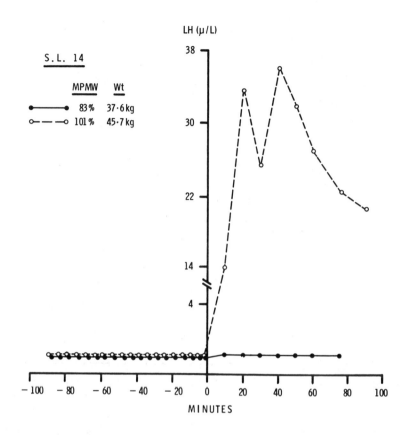

Figure 7.4. LH responses to 50 μg LHRH in males with anorexia nervosa studied during the time that they gained weight to normal (matched population mean weight) levels.

weight was 56 kg had a "normal shaped" but diminished LH response (Figure 7.5).

3. At "target" weight three subjects showed a "normal" LH response (Figures 7.5, 7.6, and 7.7). They all weighed over 60 kg. In one young subject whose target weight was only about 45 kg there was an enhanced LH response (Figure 7.4).

Finally, the FSH response to LH/RH was retained even at very low weights. It was enhanced in one subject at 45 kg and 100 percent MPMW.

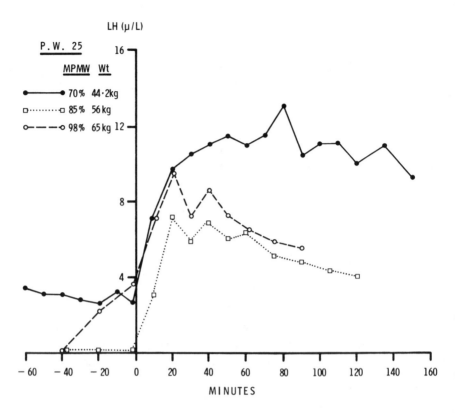

Figure 7.5. LH responses to 50 µg LHRH in males with anorexia nervosa studied during the time that they gained weight to normal (matched population mean weight) levels.

Discussion and Conclusion

Our findings of low testosterone levels that increased with weight gain but not to normal levels are in keeping with the findings reported by Beaumont, Bearwood, and Russell (1972) and of Frankel and Jenkins (1975). Previous findings on basal LH and FSH levels in the male are meager, but those that exist are in accordance with ours. Thus, Palmer, Crisp, MacKinnon, Franklin, Bonnar, & Wheeler (1975) and Frankel and Jenkins (1975) both showed a low basal LH level in one male subject which rose with refeeding. The FSH levels in both subjects bore

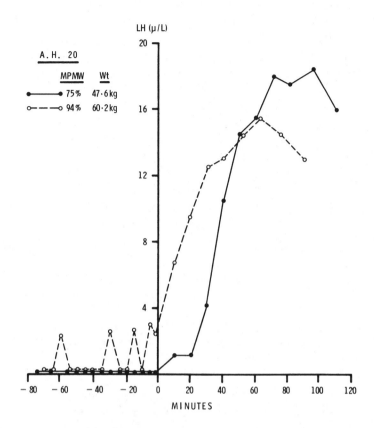

Figure 7.6. LH responses to 50 μg LHRH in males with anorexia nervosa studied during the time that they gained weight to normal (matched population mean weight) levels.

no consistent relationship with weight. Meanwhile, our basal LH and FSH findings are broadly consistent with those reported in females, that is, there is a stronger correlation with LH rather than with FSH weight (Isaacs, 1979). In our LH/RH study the LH response seems to change at different weights. At weights substantially below 45 kg there is little or no response. At around 46 ± 2 kg there seems to be an enhanced response irrespective of percentage weight. At weights substantially above 45 kg the response becomes normal. The findings on the two male subjects in the study by Palmer and co-workers (1975) and on the one subject by Frankel and Jenkins (1975) are similar to ours. In

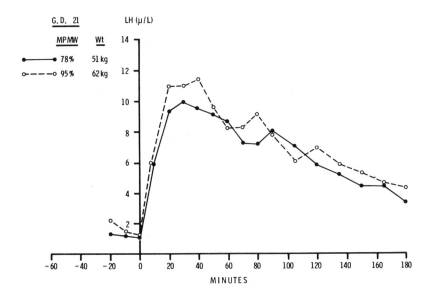

Figure 7.7. LH responses to 50 μg LHRH in males with anorexia nervosa studied during the time that they gained weight to normal (matched population mean weight) levels.

the female, Warren (1977) found that patients between 15 and 25 percent below their ideal weight showed an increased LH and FSH response to 50 μg LH/RH. Unfortunately, the actual weights and heights of their subjects were not given. Palmer and colleagues (1975) found some evidence in their females of an enhanced LH as well as FSH response to 50 μg LH/RH at around 46 kg. We merely want to indicate that this enhanced LH response in the male at around 45 kg, due perhaps to relative lack of negative feedback caused by low circulatory testosterone levels, is related more to the actual weight than the percentage MPMW of an individual. An awareness of such a threshold, with its experiential consequences for the patient, is considered important for treatment (Crisp, 1980).

References

Beaumont, P. V. J., Beardwood, C. J., & Russell, G. F. M. The occurrence of the syndrome of anorexia nervosa in male subjects. *Psychological Medicine,* 1972, *2,* 216–231.
Crisp, A. H. Anorexia nervosa. *Hospital Medicine,* 1967, *1,* 713–718.

Crisp. A. H. *Anorexia nervosa: Let me be.* London: Academic Press, 1980.

Frankel, R. J., & Jenkins, J. S. Hypothalamic-pituitary function in anorexia nervosa. *Acta endocrinology,* 1975, *78,* 209–221.

Isaacs, A. J. Endocrinology. In P. Dally, J. Gomez, & A. J. Isaacs (Eds.), *Anorexia nervosa.* London: Heinemann, 1979, pp. 158–209.

Palmer, R. L., Crisp, A. H., MacKinnon, P. C. B., Franklin, M., Bonnar, J., & Wheeler, M. Pituitary sensitivity to 50 μg LH/FSH-RH in subjects with anorexia nervosa in acute and recovery stages. *British Medical Journal,* 1975, *1,* 179–182.

Warren, M. P. Weight loss and responsiveness to LH/RH. In R. A. Vigersky (Ed.), *Anorexia nervosa.* New York: Raven Press, 1977, pp. 189–198.

8

Psychotherapy in Anorexia Nervosa and Developmental Obesity

Hilde Bruch

The treatment of anorexia nervosa and developmental obesity requires integration of various factors. There is a need for psychotherapeutic help for the severe underlying emotional and personality problems of these patients; at the same time the interactional conflicts within the family demand resolution, and the abnormal nutritional state must be corrected (Bruch, 1973, 1978).

Neither obesity nor severe undernutrition represent uniform clinical and psychiatric pictures. There are many overweight youngsters who are just that, without being emotionally disturbed. In a large group of obese children who were followed into adulthood, about one-third did fairly well, outgrew the excess weight, or remained moderately overweight, but were generally well adjusted. However, two-thirds grew progressively fatter and exhibited various degrees of maladaptation, some with severe personality problems or manifest psychiatric illness. These emotionally disturbed fat youngsters suffered excessively from the hostile social attitude, and their abnormal eating and activity patterns were recognized as intrinsically related to other disturbances of growth and maturation. In the sufferers of developmental obesity, concern with size and weight as well as inability to delay gratification or to tolerate frustration appear as central issues throughout their development.

In anorexia nervosa a distinct syndrome needs to be differentiated from various unspecific forms of psychogenic malnutrition. In the typical, primary picture *relentless pursuit of thinness* is the main issue.

This preoccupation with size can be recognized as a final step in a desperate struggle for a sense of control and the achievement of personal identity and effectiveness. This struggle usually has gone on in various disguises for some time. Perfectionistic academic performance and excellence in athletics are common early manifestations. In these patients the term *anorexia* is a misnomer; they do not suffer from true loss of appetite. On the contrary, they experience tormenting hunger pains, though they may deny it during the illness and confess it only much later, and like other starving people they are frantically preoccupied with food and eating. The self-starvation is strenuously maintained with the goal of obtaining the ultimate in thinness. In the atypical forms, the eating function itself is disturbed and food is endowed with various threatening meanings. The weight loss is incidental to this avoidance of food and often complained of, or valued only for its coercive effect, in contrast to the pride with which the true anorexic defends her skeleton-like appearance as beautiful or delusionally denies the emaciation. These atypical cases vary considerably in the severity of illness and accessibility to treatment. I shall limit my discussion here to the psychotherapeutic problems encountered in developmental obesity and primary anorexia nervosa, which appear to be on the increase.

Psychodynamic Diagnosis

It is common practice to rate the severity of obesity and anorexia nervosa in terms of the weight deviation—in absolute figures or as percentage deviation from the norm. In anorexia nervosa this figure is supplemented by references to amenorrhea, constipation, dry skin, and so forth. These measurements describe the visible aspects of the clinical picture, but contribute little to the understanding of the underlying psychologic problems. Though anorexia nervosa and developmental obesity look like extreme opposites, they have many features in common. In both conditions severe disturbances in body image and self-concept are prominent; food intake and body size are manipulated in a misguided effort to solve or camouflage inner stress or adjustment difficulties. These youngsters do not feel identified with their bodies, but look upon the body as an external object over which they must exercise rigid control (anorexia nervosa) or in relation to which they feel helpless (obesity with its lack of will power). Though stubbornness and negativism are conspicuous in the clinical picture, these youngsters suffer behind this facade from a devastating sense of ineffectiveness;

they feel powerless to control their bodies and also to direct their lives in general. They experience themselves as empty and lacking in the sense of ownership of their own bodies and as controlled by others. They are helpless and ineffective in all their functioning, not self-directed or truly separated from others. They act and behave as if they were the misshapen and wrong product of somebody else's actions, as if their center of gravity was not within themselves. They lack discriminating awareness of bodily needs; specifically, they are unable to recognize hunger and satiety. They also fail to identify other states of bodily discomfort such as cold or fatigue, or to discriminate bodily tensions from anxiety, depression, or other psychological stresses.

These deficits in the sense of ownership and control of the body color the way obese and anorexic youngsters face their problems of living, their relationships to others, and in particular the problems of approaching adolescence. Like other youngsters they must prepare themselves for self-sufficiency and independence and emancipate themselves from the dependency on their mothers and families, but they are poorly equipped for these tasks. Not infrequently they have been overprotected, overcontrolled, and overvalued, with few experiences outside the home, so that adolescence with the need to grow beyond the family attitudes and values becomes a threatening demand. The parents, in their dissatisfaction with themselves and each other, have invested great expectations in them to compensate for their own frustrations. Frequently these youngsters feel deprived of the support and recognition from their peers which help normal adolescents in this process of liberation. Recognition of these deficits is not always easy because these problems are overshadowed by the visible symptoms and the struggle over food, which is conducted with mutual blame and increasing rage. The obese when unable to adhere to a diet is condemned as greedy and weak-willed, and the anorexic's refusal to eat is experienced and responded to as a hostile attack on or rejection of the parents.

Conceptual Model of Early Development

Inability to eat normally sets fat and anorexic youngsters apart. Traditional psychoanalysis has explained this as resulting from the attachment of sexual and aggressive impulses to the hunger drive. My own observations led to the conclusion that hunger awareness is not innate knowledge, but that it requires for its proper organization early learning experiences that may be correct or incorrect, depending upon whether the responses of the food giver fit the child's needs. Detailed reconstruction of the essential early experiences of these patients revealed that expression of the child's needs has been disregarded or inappropriately responded to. Characteristically, they had been given adequate, even excellent, physical care, but it had been superimposed according to the mother's concepts instead of being geared to the clues given by the child.

A simplified model of interactional patterns was constructed, with the assumption that from birth onward two basic forms of behavior need to be differentiated, namely, behavior that is *initiated* in the infant and behavior in *response* to stimuli; this distinction applies to both the biological and the social psychological field. Behavior in relation to the child can be described as *responsive* or *stimulating,* and the interaction can be rated as *appropriate* or *inappropriate* depending on whether it fits the need expressed by the child.

Appropriate responses to clues coming from the infant are essential for the organization of his initially diffuse urges into differentiated patterns of self-awareness, competence, and effectiveness. If confirmation and reinforcement of expression of his needs and impulses are absent, contradictory, or inaccurate, then the child will grow up perplexed when trying to identify disturbances in his biological fields or to differentiate them from emotional and interpersonal disturbances. He will be apt to misinterpret deformities in his self-body concept as externally induced, and he will be deficient in his sense of separateness and experience his body image in a distorted way. He will be passive and helpless under the influence of internal urges or external forces. These features are also characteristic of schizophrenia. This developmental scheme offers a clue to the close association of severe eating disorders and schizophrenic development.

The reconstructed early feeding histories are often conspicuous by their blandness, particularly in anorexia nervosa. The parents stress that the patient has been unusually good as a child, never giving any trouble or fussing about food, eating exactly what was put before him. If the mother's concepts are not out of line with a child's physiological needs, everything may look normal on the surface. Obesity in a child may be a measure of a mother's overestimation of his needs or of her using food indiscriminately as a universal pacifier. The gross deficits in initiative and active self-awareness, the lack of inner controls, including the inability to regulate the food intake, become manifest only when the child is confronted with new situations and demands, for which the misleading routine of his early life has left him unprepared. Not having developed an integrated self and body concept, he will feel helpless when confronted with the biological, social and psychological demands of adolescence. If every tension is experienced as "need to eat," instead of arousing anxiety, anger, or other appropriate emotions, he will become progressively obese. The anorexic tries to compensate for this deficit in inner controls in an exaggerated way by denying the need for sufficient food. The manifest clinical picture may develop under the stress of puberty itself; in others only at times of additional new demands, such as entering a new school, separation from home, or when a reducing regimen is rigidly enforced.

Psychotherapeutic Intervention

These theoretical considerations are the outcome of continuous reevaluation of the therapeutic results, in particular of the failure of the traditional psychoanalytic approach. The literature on the value of psychoanalysis for the treatment of eating disorders is hopelessly inconclusive, and clarification was not possible until distinct pictures were described. Authors with extensive experience with true anorexia nervosa and also developmental obesity recognized early that conventional psychoanalytic explanations did not apply to these patients and that psychoanalytic treatment was ineffective. My own investigations of the therapeutic situation as a transactional process led to the conclusion that the classic psychoanalytic setting, where the patient expresses his secret thoughts and feelings and the analyst interprets their unconscious meaning, contains for patients with eating disorders elements that represent the painful repetition of patterns that had characterized their whole development, namely of being told by someone else what they feel and how to think, with the implication that they are incapable of doing it themselves. The profound sense of ineffectiveness that has troubled them all their lives is thus confirmed and reinforced. The essential task of the therapeutic intervention must be correction of this deficit by offering patients assistance in developing awareness of their capabilities and potentials and thus helping them to become more competent to handle their problems of living in less painful and less ineffective ways. These modifications are in good agreement with modern concepts of psychotherapy that have been developed for the treatment of schizophrenia, borderline states, and narcissistic personalities. To meet the needs of such patients, special consideration must be given to the deficits in their sense of autonomy and to their disturbed self-concept and self-awareness.

The approach to obesity and anorexia nervosa, even of experienced therapists, seems to have remained tied to ineffective and outmoded concepts, such as considering the psychological disorder as the outcome of oral dependency, incorporative cannibalism, rejection or pregnancy fantasies, or similar unconscious conflicts. With the new formulation, the therapeutic focus is on the patient's failure in self-experience, on his defective tools and concepts for organizing and expressing his needs, and on his bewilderment in dealing with others. Therapy represents an attempt to repair the conceptual defects and distortions, the deep-seated dissatisfaction and sense of isolation, and the underlying sense of incompetence.

The therapist's task is to be alert and consistent in recognizing any self-initiated behavior and expressions on the part of the patient. To do so the therapist needs to pay minute attention to the discrepancies in the patient's recall of the past and to the way the patient misperceives or misinterprets current events to which he will then respond inappropriately; and the therapist must be honest in confirming or correcting what the patient communicates. When held to a detailed examination of the when, where, who, and how, real or fantasied difficulties and emotional stresses will come into focus and the patient will discover the problems hidden behind the facade of his abnormal eating behavior.

Although inability to identify bodily sensations correctly is the specific disability in eating disorders, other feeling tones are inaccurately perceived or conceptualized. These patients suffer from an abiding sense of loneliness, or from the feeling of not being respected by others, and this is related to the inability to recognize interpersonal implications. They often feel insulted and abused, though the realistic situation may not contain these elements. The anticipation or recall of a real or imagined insult may lead to withdrawal from the actual situation and flight into an eating binge—or to reinforcement of the self-starvation. Exploration of the realistic aspects of these experiences, and examination of alternatives in such situations, eventually helps a patient to experience himself not as utterly helpless or as a victim of a compulsion that overpowers him, but as increasingly competent to deal realistically with problems. Having functioned as an active participant in the treatment process, and with increasing awareness of impulses, feelings, and needs originating within himself, he will learn to recognize appropriate feelings and reactions in areas of functioning where he had been deprived of adequate early learning. Gradually, he becomes more competent to live his life as a self-directed, authentic individual who is capable of enjoying what life has to offer.

Under this approach even patients who had been unsuccessfully in treatment for several years and who were filled to the brim with useless, though not necessarily incorrect, knowledge of their psychodynamics will begin to change and then relinquish their self-punishing rituals. The important point is that patients learn to examine their own development in realistic terms, with emphasis on their own contributions or on defining the areas in which they had felt excluded from active participation. Examining their own development in this way becomes an important stimulus for acquiring thus far deficient mental tools and for a repair of their cognitive distortions; they learn to rely upon their own thinking and can become more realistic in their self-appraisal.

This approach implies a definite change in the therapist's concept of his role, and it is not always easy to make this change. It involves permitting a patient to express what he experiences without immediately explaining or labeling it; in other words, it requires suspending one's assumed knowledge and expertise. Some of the current models of psychiatric training emphasize early formulation of the underlying psychodynamic issues, but this formulation may then stand in the way of learning the truly relevant facts. A therapist who assumes that he understands the patient's problem is not quite so alert and curious in unraveling the unclear and confused periods. He may be tempted to superimpose his prematurely conceived notions on the patient or become preoccupied with what he will find, whether it confirms his assumptions, instead of engaging the patient in becoming a collaborator in the search for unknown factors. It is important that a therapist recognize meaningful messages in seeming generalities that are often labeled as evasive; never having experienced confirmation for anything they expressed, these patients, though often unusually gifted, can verbalize their state of profound bewilderment only through such stereotyped complaints.

Part of the therapeutic role is to make it possible for patients to uncover their own abilities, resources, and inner capacities for thinking, judging, and feeling, and they will respond well when they recognize the therapist's fact-finding attitude, that he does not have some secret knowledge that he withholds from them. Once the capacity of self-recognition has been experienced, there is usually a change in the whole atmosphere of involvement in the treatment process.

In spite of the overt negativistic attitude, these patients are unusually alert to what is going on, and indications of some change may become apparent in the first few sessions, namely, when they recognize that what they have to say is listened to as important. Instead of focusing on the motives underlying the overeating or noneating, I find it useful to inquire about their general development in the spirit of getting acquainted, about their feelings of self-confidence and satisfaction with themselves. Most will reply that they never had confidence in themselves, that they had lived by doing only what was expected of them. Some will name a definite event that made them aware that something was wrong with their way of life.

To give just one example, Joyce was nearly 18 years old when she and her parents came for consultation. She had been anorexic for two and a half years and she, and also her parents, had been in treatment throughout this period, with two hospitalizations to enforce weight gain. However, her weight was only 32 kg (height 165 cm). In the expectation that she would again be exposed to a weight-gaining regimen, she had lost 5 kg during the month preceding the consultation. She was an only child born to middle-aged parents who were deeply devoted to her and had encouraged all her unusual intellectual and artistic talents. As the consultation progressed it was recognized that this very giftedness and success in all undertakings had left Joyce with a depleted sense of value, that this was what she owed her parents who enjoyed and cherished her successes. Unless an activity required great effort and strain she rated it as "ordinary" and of no value to her; only the "eccentric," or extraordinary, gave her a feeling of worthwhileness in her own right.

During the first session in which the parents participated, Joyce mentioned that she felt the true onset of her illness had occurred much earlier, when she was about 12 years old; while having tea her mother warned her not to take a third cookie. When this was taken up during the next session, the parents shrugged it off as one of her attempts to blame them for her illness. Joyce had mentioned this episode to her previous therapists, who had called it "intellectualizing" or who had paid no attention to it. She definitely felt this episode was important though she did not know why. To my question of whether she might have become aware at that moment that mother had control over her body and told her what she needed because she did not trust Joyce to rely on her own sensations and judgment, she smiled for the first time and asked: "Is that why I get so angry when Father tells me I am tired?"

From then on she appeared like a changed person who spoke freely about her long-standing anguish that nothing was her own, that she had felt obliged to live her whole life as her parents had planned it; in particular she had been horrified about having to lead the life of a teenager to satisfy them. This issue had not come up at all with her former therapists, whom she described as having been silent and expecting her to keep on talking, and who would then tell her what it meant. She never felt that they were right or that it mattered what they said. Within a few sessions she openly expressed that up to now she had resisted the idea of "getting well" because this had meant only having weight put on her and being told what to think and how to behave. For the first time she was confident that therapy might help her in becoming her own person and to be someone individual.

What a patient offers as a vital issue varies, of course, from case to case. The important point is that seemingly ordinary, even silly memories are taken seriously and then used as a meaningful explanation of the illness, which may be defined as a fight against the feeling of nothingness or ruthless punishment for not living up to expectations. Having never trusted themselves to acknowledge their own needs, these patients need to experience in therapy that they have the right to express and pursue their own wants and wishes.

Once patients feel understood and respected in their deepest concerns and experience that the therapist follows their lead about important issues, they are more apt to listen to his or her explanations and to realize that meaningful psychotherapy is not possible as long as they are in the state of acute starvation, since that in itself makes their psychological reactions abnormal; that the cadaverous appearance arouses strong reactions in others that interfere with all human relationships; and that the therapist's anxious concern about it might interfere with the progress of treatment, since this places undue emphasis on physical status instead of on the causative factors of illness. Once rapport has been established, a patient is willing to accept that the problems that precipitated the whole illness will remain inaccessible to clarification as long as the nutrition is abnormally low. Thus they will come to the point of permitting the weight to rise gradually, without experiencing a loss of self-esteem and pride, and become capable of facing the problems of increasing independence, autonomy, and maturity.

Family Involvement

There are few conditions that arouse so much frustration, alarm, panic, anger, rage, and mutual blame as the spectacle of a starving child stubbornly refusing to eat or vomiting what has been taken in. One might say that paradoxically a "low weight" carries much weight in the family. Though less dramatic, but usually of longer duration, in obesity too all family concerns seem to focus on what the patient eats and weighs. Meaningful therapy is not possible unless the fighting forces are disengaged. A series of enthusiastic recent reports have dealt with crisis-oriented family intervention with immediate changes in the ongoing patterns of interaction. They usually deal with young patients, in the beginning of the illness, before the complicating secondary problems have become entrenched. Thus far there have been no reports about the long-term value of these dramatic rearrangements. They are not without dangers; the possibility of serious suicide attempts and psychotic disorganization must be kept in mind.

The therapeutic involvement of a family needs to be conceived of as occurring in several phases. Resolving the acute conflicts over the eating is necessary, but it alone is not enough. To recognize and resolve the lifelong patterns of interaction is of even greater importance, since they have resulted in this abnormal development of a youngster without a competent sense of identity. In anorexia nervosa the surface picture is often that of a smoothly functioning family; however, underlying the apparent marital harmony there is often a deep sense of disappointment with each other, with the patient feeling obliged to compensate for this. The overintense involvement with one or the other parent often expresses the parent's own need for closeness. Clarifying this enmeshment requires that the parents acknowledge their own problems, which they need to resolve in grown-up terms by finding comfort in each other. This is a prerequisite for patients' becoming liberated from the bondage, free to pursue their own life as a basic right.

The need for family therapy has become widely accepted, but unfortunately it is often carried out without recognizable benefit. Though a family has met regularly, over a considerable period of time, with a therapist, a positive understanding of each other may not be achieved, namely, when the focus is only on the family's shortcomings, or the sole recommendation is a hands-off policy. One patient described it as: "He would just sit there and we would argue and fight and lash out in a kind of raw anger, but nothing would get accomplished. We never listened to each other, and he did not help us to recognize what the others were saying." She contrasted this with a helpful experience during which the excessive mutual concern was pointed out as a problem, with each one taking over the feelings and goals of the others. The emphasis was on the loving aspects of the family interaction, which gave them a sense of confidence that there was something positive to work for.

No general outline can be given of how best to conduct work with families and how to combine it with individual psychotherapy; the focus, length, and intensity will vary considerably in different cases. Whether a patient can be treated effectively while living at home depends to a large extent on whether the family conflicts are handled successfully. Hospitalization may be necessary, not only to effect a weight gain, but also to institute psychotherapy and to clarify the underlying family problems in the absence of the patient. Treating only the patient while hospitalized, without involving the family, will nearly unavoidably result in a relapse when the patient rejoins the family group.

Weight Change

For effective and lasting correction of the abnormal body weight, the dietary program must be coordinated with psychotherapy and resolution of the family conflicts. All too often the abnormal weight is approached as an isolated symptom, and weight loss or gain is enforced from the outside. An unending stream of publications report successful dietary treatment, but rarely with information on the long-term results. The psychiatrist is apt to see the failures of this simplistic approach.

In obesity it will depend upon the severity of the condition whether and when to recommend a reducing program. Viewed as a manipulation of the energy balance, treatment of obesity is simple; reduction of food intake and increase in exercise accomplishes a predictable loss in weight or stabilization at a desirable level. Commonly, mothers are instructed about such dietary restrictions. The more important task would be to teach them how to recognize a child's real needs and how to encourage him or her to find satisfaction other than through food. Characteristically fat children are passive, immature, and helpless, and a dietary regimen should help them develop the capacity for inner controls instead of being something superimposed by others. This is of particular importance for adolescents who will diet only when it is a challenge to their initiative and responsibility.

In anorexia nervosa correcting the abnormal weight is often a matter of great urgency; the very survival of a youngster may be at stake. There have been continuous debates on how to accomplish the seemingly impossible task of getting food into patients who are stubbornly determined to starve themselves. As in obesity, the physiological principles are simple: increase the intake and restrict the activities of these starving but hyperactive youngsters.

Recently, behavior modification has been described with great enthusiasm as a method that guarantees rapid increase in weight. The first report by Stunkard and Mahoney (1976) recommended freely chosen activities as a reward for gaining weight. One of their four patients with satisfactory weight gain committed suicide after discharge. The method has since been refined by permitting access to all kinds of desirable activities only as a "reinforcement" for weight gain. It appears that with this approach faster gain in weight is achieved than with any other method. However, the long-term results dramatically illustrate that weight gain in itself is not a cure for anorexia nervosa. I have observed catastrophic long-range effects in a series of patients previously treated with behavior modification. Serious depression, psychotic disorganization, and suicide attempts follow this method of weight gain so often that it must be considered dangerous. Without psychological support and help toward better self-understanding, this method undermines the last vestiges of self-esteen and destroys the crucial hope of ever achieving autonomy and self-determination.

It is equally dangerous not to correct the weight and to permit a patient to exist at a marginal level of safety. This error is not uncommonly committed by psychotherapists in the unrealistic hope that once the underlying unconscious conflicts are recognized, the whole picture will correct itself. Sometimes years are spent in a futile effort, precious time is lost, and patients stay excluded from the necessary experiences of the adolescent years. The starvation itself has such a distorting effect on all psychic functioning that no true picture of the psychological problems can be formulated until the worst malnutrition is corrected. Only then will important underlying problems become accessible to therapy. The same applies to the handling of binge eating and vomiting, which may have become habitual by the time a psychiatrist is consulted. Without interrupting this behavior, for which hospitalization may become necessary, the basic problems, in particular the fear of emptiness, loneliness, and conviction of helplessness, cannot be clarified. A passive attitude on the part of the therapist implies that he condones the abnormal behavior, which camouflages the underlying psychological issues, and treatment may be unnecessarily prolonged.

Conclusion

Anorexia nervosa and juvenile obesity have the reputation of offering unusual treatment difficulties, and relapses or outright failures are not uncommon. This appears to be related to erroneous or inconsistent treatment efforts. Results are closely linked to the pertinence of the psychodynamic understanding, and the pursuit of meaningful treatment goals. If the unrealistic expectations with which so many obese youngsters approach dieting remain uncorrected or, worse, if the therapist shares them, the outcome may well be the repeated sad cycle of frantic reducing and even more rapid regaining. However, with realistic goals, focused on achieving a more competent, less painful way of handling problems of living, including the ability to establish weight control at a reasonable level, the long-range treatment results are surprisingly good. Progress needs to be evaluated not only as weight stability, but also in terms of adequacy of living. Those fat youngsters who had gained insight into the underlying problems achieved a high level of functioning, were successful in their work, got married, and functioned adequately as marriage partners and parents. They raised their children with good control over their eating, so that they grew up slim, not plagued by excess weight like the parent.

In anorexia nervosa the relationship of treatment success to the pertinence of the approach is even more apparent. Though early institution of a meaningful, comprehensive therapeutic program improves the chances of recovery, long-standing illness does not preclude good results, even after many years of futile effort, as long as underlying lack of autonomy is made the focus of therapy. Evaluating the long-range outcome has led to the conclusion that no one factor of the clinical picture is predictive of success or failure; rather, all factors are directly related to the competence and adequacy of the therapeutic intervention and its integration with nutritional restitution and correction of the faulty patterns of family interaction.

References

Bruch, H. *Eating disorders: Obesity, anorexia nervosa, and the person within.* New York: Basic Books, 1973.

Bruch, H. *The golden cage: The enigma of anorexia nervosa.* Cambridge: Harvard University Press, 1978.

Stunkard, A. J., & Mahoney, M. J. Behavioral treatment of eating disorders. In H. Leitenberg (Ed.), *The handbook of behavior modification.* Englewood Cliffs, N.J.: Prentice-Hall, 1976.

9

Sleep, Eating, and Weight Disorders

Frederick J. Evans

We sleep for about one-third of our lives, and a significant portion of our waking activities are concerned with food intake: its collection, preparation, and the social customs and rituals associated with it. These vegetative functions are an important part of human activity, but they are often taken for granted. The likelihood that sleep and eating might produce complex interactions has been considered by only a small number of scientists. Before discussing the relationship between sleep, eating, and weight, it is necessary to summarize some relevant background knowledge about sleep.

Normal Sleep:
An Overview

Historically, sleep was considered a period of passivity that had no special significance except for those psychodynamically oriented psychiatrists interested in dreaming. In the 1963 revision of his 1939 book, Kleitman reviewed more than 4,000 articles on sleep, many of them showing sophisticated clinical and observational insights into the relationship between sleep, eating, and weight disorders. However, it was the development of the EEG classification of stages of sleep, and

I wish to thank Erica Bergstrom, Barbara Marcelo Evans, Richard Goodstein, Cyril M. Franks, R. Lynn Horne, Lawrence Klein, Helen M. Pettinati, Joanne Rosenberg, A. Arthur Sugerman, George Wilson, and particularly Julie Staats for their helpful comments. This review was supported by the Carrier Foundation Division of Research. Because of the important gaps in knowledge in this area, the aim of this review is to be provocative, even if occasionally wrong, rather than encyclopedic.

the later somewhat fortuitous discovery (Aserinsky & Kleitman, 1953) of the relationship between a certain physiological stage of sleep (the rapid eye movement or REM stage) and its association with a high incidence of dream recall (Dement & Kleitman, 1957) that stimulated the tremendous interest that sleep has held for scientists of many disciplines over the last 25 years.

EEG Stages of Sleep

Sleep is a highly organized structural phenomenon that does not consist of a single unitary biological and physiological state. Several distinct stages, shown in Figure 9.1, cycle predictably throughout the night.

The typical EEG pattern of the resting, eyes-closed adult shows epochs of EEG occipital alpha activity (7 to 13 cps) intermixed with bursts of high-voltage fast activity, which predominates in the *resting waking* record. As the alpha become desynchronized, the person produces a fast, flat EEG that is the drowsy, sleep onset *stage 1*. Sleep is usually not considered to be present until the emergence of lower-amplitude sleep spindles of 14 to 16 cps (mostly in the frontal regions), usually accompanied by K-complexes; this is *stage 2*. After a few minutes, large-amplitude 1 to 4 cps delta waves appear. This is a deep restorative sleep and is called *stage 3 to 4, delta, or slow wave sleep* (SWS). After about 90 minutes of delta and stage 2 cycling, a dramatic change occurs, not only in the EEG channels, but in several associated systems. Following a body movement, the EEG emerges as a fast desynchronized record that cannot easily be detected from the EEG of the active alert waking state. The eyes are moving quite rapidly, in much the way that they might if they were scanning a scene, but the person is still asleep because there are no eye blinks in this record (for the eyes are indeed closed) and the body muscles are totally relaxed—for example, the chin EMG reaches its most flaccid level of the whole night. This is called *REM sleep* (or paradoxical sleep in animals). If awakened from sleep during REM, the person almost invariably reports a dream. However, if awakened at any other point during the night, the chances of a dream report are quite low.

Although the initial REM period is relatively short (often less than five minutes), the REM phase appears again, about every 90 minutes in adults, becoming progressively longer, until by the end of the night it occupies most of sleeping time. In young adults, about 22 percent of the average night is spent in REM sleep, about 25 percent in slow-wave sleep, and the remainder (about 50 percent) in stage 2.

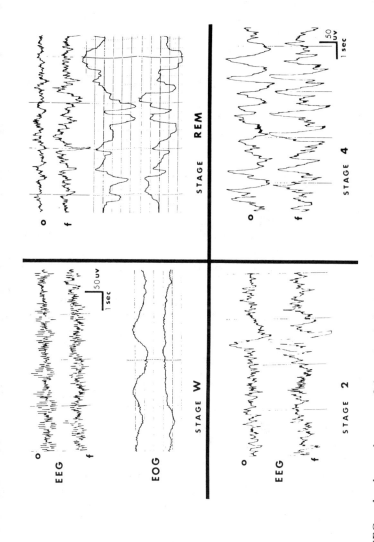

Figure 9.1. EEG and polygraph stages of sleep. Typical EEG patterns are shown for stage 2 and stage 4 (SWS); horizontal eye-movement patterns are also included for eyes closed, relaxed waking, and REM stage.

Adapted from a figure previously published in F. J. Evans, Hypnosis and sleep. In E. Fromm & R. E. Shor (Eds.), *Hypnosis*. New York: Aldine, 1972 (1st ed.), pp. 63–83; 1979 (revised 2nd ed.), pp. 139–183.

The average young adult has a sleep-onset latency of about 20 minutes, total sleep time (TST) of seven and a half hours, and two or three transient awakenings during the night. While there are marked individual differences in sleep length, the percentage distribution of the stages during normal uninterrupted sleep remains relatively constant. The percentage of REM sleep is greater in early childhood. The percent of SWS diminishes rapidly in the elderly and is often absent in depressed patients.

Although stage 2 sleep predominates, virtually nothing is known of its nature and functions. It is elastic: when changes occur in the amount of REM and SWS sleep, they are compensated for by corresponding changes in stage 2.

Selective Sleep
Deprivation and REM Rebound

We are only too well aware from our personal lives of the subjective and emotional effects of sleep deprivation. However, these effects have been proven to be most resistant to documentation in the laboratory, partly because long-term sleep deprivation is impossible—eventually, we fall asleep! When we lose sleep, a sleep debt builds up which must be paid back. However, within broad limits, we need make up only some of the sleep we lose.

The functions of REM and SWS have been investigated by selective sleep-deprivation studies. Subjects can be awakened whenever they are in SWS or REM, but not stage 2 sleep (which would involve total sleep deprivation). Uninterrupted recovery sleep can then be studied. In general, SWS takes priority in recovery from sleep deprivation, but the recovery of REM sleep is more dramatic. Following sleep loss or REM sleep reduction, REM occurs sooner than after the usual 90 minutes, and REM can account for almost 30 percent compared with the usual 22 percent of the night's sleep. This is the so-called *REM rebound effect*. After extensive sleep loss, REM typically takes at least three to five days to return to baseline levels. During REM rebound, sleep is often more fragmented, and the increased frequency of REM periods and REM length, as well as the consequent anxiety-laden dreams and nightmares that typically occur, contribute to a dysphoric mood upon awakening. The anxiety, restless sleep, fatigue, and mood changes are probably partly responsible for the continued use of barbiturates and other REM-suppressing drugs, since the consequences of voluntary attempts to withdraw are perceived as much more negative than any positive effects erroneously attributed to the continued ingestion of the drug.

REM sleep is a highly activated state. Although muscle tonicity is extremely flaccid, peaks of biochemical, physiological, and psychological activity occur during REM. REM is associated with variability in heart rate, respiration, and blood pressure, rises in plasma and urinary hydroxycorticosteroid levels, and increased firing rates of individual neurons. Rapid middle-ear and throat muscle vibrations, penile erections, and vaginal excitation occur and may signal the onset of REM. Indeed, the internal system is in a state of physiological turmoil, protected by the superstructure of the relaxation of the peripheral musculature. It is, therefore, not entirely surprising that the incidence of myocardial infarctions, cerebral accidents, seizure activity, and asthmatic and duodenal ulcer attacks have a higher incidence during REM sleep than at any other time during the 24-hour period. Rapid withdrawal from the many medications that suppress REM or produce REM rebound on withdrawal (Kay, Blackburn, Buckingham, & Karacan, 1976) could conceivably place at medical risk patients prone to such diseases.

Sleep Satisfaction and
Changes in Sleep Patterns

Whether reduction in REM sleep caused by sleep-onset insomnia, frequent nighttime awakenings, restless sleep, and truncated sleep due to early morning awakenings subsequently produce the same unpleasant REM rebound consequences found following drug-induced REM suppression has not been firmly established. Little is known of the relationship between sleep satisfaction and the order, integrity, and percentage of sleep stages (Johnson, 1973). Napping studies have shown that satisfaction is related to the amount of SWS sleep (Dinges, Orne, Orne, & Evans, 1980) and that at least with habitual nappers (Lawrence, 1971), naps containing REM sleep are perceived as unpleasant. This is probably the reason why habitual nappers avoid REM sleep by typically napping for less than 90 minutes (the usual latency to first REM)—a point not previously recognized in the sleep literature. Sleep satisfaction may turn out to relate to percent REM time in a U-shaped function: too much or too little may lead to dysphoric mood. Thus, while not definitively proven, temporary sleep stage truncation and specific stage rebound effects due to transient reductions in SWS or REM may produce negative psychological effects.

General Metabolic and
Anabolic Processes during Sleep

Although specific functions of sleep and its stages are not understood, it is widely held (though poorly documented) that SWS serves anabolic and restorative functions. Germane to this topic is the recent hypothesis that REM sleep is related to increased protein synthesis (Adam & Oswald, 1977a, b; Rojas-Ramirez, Shkurovich, Ugartechea, & Drucker-Colin, 1976). This hypothesis would comfortably encompass the more popular view that REM is related to information processing and the transfer and consolidation from short-term to long-term memory storage.

Several changes associated with both REM and SWS may have significance in understanding the relationship between nutrition and sleep, particularly in terms of understanding some of the metabolic and anabolic processes involved. Danguir and Nicolaidis (1979) found that food restitution or the infusion of glucose up to 100 percent of normal daily caloric intake in severely starved rats led to a dramatic rebound in both the SWS and the REM sleep that had been decreased during the food deprivation. Hall, Orr, and Stahl (1976) showed that following the feeding of liquid meals, gastric emptying and acid-secretion functions during sleep accelerate during REM sleep in normal subjects. Gastric contractions are not related to sleep stages (Kleitman, Mullin, Cooperman, & Titelbaum, 1937; Lavie, Kripke, Hiatt, & Harrison, 1978), though they may be related to body motility during sleep.

Sitarim, Moore, and Gillin (1978) suggest that the normal dietary constituent choline might be involved in the regulation of REM latency and REM percentages during the night. The correlation between initial placebo effect and change in REM after choline was $-.9$ ($N = 12$, $p < .01$). Pavlinac, Berman, Kripke, and Deftos (1978) reported that both parathyroid hormone and calcium concentrations in plasma were significantly related to REM sleep. Kripke, Lavie, Parker, Huey, and Deftos (1978) showed that plasma parathyroid hormone and plasma calcium levels were related, respectively, to SWS and REM cycles. Mendelson, Slater, Gold, and Gillin (1980) have expanded earlier studies showing that growth hormone release induces increases in REM sleep and possible decreases in SWS. They showed that injections of growth hormone 15 minutes before bedtime led to a 19 percent decrease in SWS and a 13 percent increase in REM sleep ($p < .01, p < .05$, respectively in 18 young adults), even though total sleep time was not changed.

No attempt will be made to integrate diverse metabolic and biochemical changes, such as in the sampling above and others summarized below, since sufficient replicated data are not yet available. This sampling suggests the extreme complexities involved in sleep, eating, and weight interactions.

Changes in Sleep during Weight Gain and Loss

When a person experiences sudden changes in weight, corresponding changes in sleep patterns are typically observed. In general, any sudden increase in weight tends to be associated with an increase in total sleep time. Sudden weight loss is typically associated with a decrease in total sleep time, increased body motility, and disturbed and unsatisfying sleep.

The relationship between weight loss and sleep changes has been most convincingly demonstrated in animal studies. Jacobs and McGinty (1971) showed that the less food rats received, the less they slept. After six to 11 days of food deprivation, virtually all sleep disappeared. In animal studies, the effects of dramatic weight loss are most clearly evident in increased activity levels. For example, Treichler and Hall (1962) found that activity levels of rats increased by 1,400 percent when a starvation diet had reduced the animals to 60 percent of original body weight. Activity during total starvation in rats increased until weakness intervened after about four days.

In human neonates, Kleitman (1963) showed that the 50- to 60-minute rest–activity cycle of the neonate soon becomes coupled with the three- to four-hour gastric motility and feeding cycle.

The relationship between eating and sleep behavior is quite obvious in free-roaming animals: there is survival value to a food/sleep association. While the starving animal is increasingly forced to forgo sleep to forage for food, the satiated animal is probably safest if it can sleep and remain camouflaged between food-seeking forays. Indeed, Webb (1975) has argued that this is precisely the evolutionary significance of sleep. Sleep protects the animal between feedings from predators. He argues, with considerable empirical support (see review by Dinges et al., 1980), that fragmented sleep throughout the 24-hour period is probably more beneficial than the modern eight hours of continuous nighttime sleep.

Information regarding the relationship between weight change and changes in sleep in human adults comes mainly from the psychiatric literature. Regardless of diagnosis, there is a positive correlation between weight loss and disturbed or reduced sleep, on the one hand, and weight gain and increased sleep on the other (Crisp & Stonehill, 1976). This relationship is found most frequently in anorexia nervosa patients and will be discussed below. Separate from the anorexia literature, a number of studies (Beck, 1967; Carney, Roth, & Garside, 1965; Kiloh & Garside, 1963; Michaelis, 1964) have documented the relationship between insomnia and weight loss. A correlation of .23 ($p <$ .01) was found between early morning awakenings and weight loss in 129 depressed inpatients (Carney et al., 1965). A similar correlation was found in an outpatient population (Kiloh & Garside, 1963). The triad of loss of appetite, weight loss, and insomnia are standard defining characteristics of endogenous depression.

The mechanisms whereby food intake should be related to sleep are at best speculative at this stage. When milk or fat is directly introduced into the duodenum of cats, sleep is enhanced (Fara, Rubinstein, & Sonnenschien, 1969). These researchers postulated that a gastrointestinal hormone or an indirect neurogenic mechanism is triggered through the stimulation of duodenal receptors. The role of tryptophan as a mediator will be discussed below. Kales and Kales (1974) have suggested links through thyroid functioning. Hypothyroidism results in weight gain and long sleep, with a relative absence of SWS, whereas hyperthyroidism is associated with weight loss and short intensive sleep, with a relative increase in the amount of SWS. It is interesting to note that a blunted thyroid-stimulating hormone response to infusion of thyroid-releasing hormone has recently been implicated in the prediction of the course of unipolar depression (Gold, Pottash, Davies, Ryan, Sweeney, & Martin, 1979). Sleep disturbances in these patients were not discussed, but were presumably present.

The older literature (reviewed by Kleitman, 1963) suggests that body movement and (hunger-related) stomach contractions occur simultaneously during sleep. Wada (1922) and Laird and Drexel (1934) discovered body motility increased following hard-to-digest diets of food containing hemicellulose compared to relatively easy-to-digest food (such as cornflakes and milk) given as bedtime snacks. Body motility was used as a (somewhat unreliable) measure of restless sleep/nighttime awakening prior to the development of EEG technology. If dieting increases stomach contractions, it seems likely that motility would increase, possibly signifying poor sleep.

If weight loss produces increased activity and increased nighttime sleep motility, it is important to note that moderate exercise will have a detrimental or beneficial effect on sleep depending on its timing in relationship to sleep onset. Engaging in exercise less than two to three hours before sleep is likely to impair sleep onset and to produce a reduction in SWS. Moderate exercise performed at least two hours before bedtime is often reported to improve the quality of sleep, reduce motility, and increase SWS. Therapeutically, these results suggest that if a successful weight-reducing program is to avoid producing sleep difficulties, it should be accompanied by appropriate regulation of the increased activity level so that activity is minimized in the period before bed. Moderate exercise more than two hours before bedtime and an easy-to-digest (high tryptophan) bedtime snack has been suggested (but not documented) as an aid in weight-loss programs.

The importance of a bedtime snack in the elderly is underscored by the hypoglycemia that may occur during the nighttime fast. This may be accentuated by the "tea and toast" nutritional irregularity often encountered in the elderly living alone. Inadequate regulation of blood-sugar levels may lead to glycosuria and nocturia in elderly diabetics. Adjustment of the diabetic regimen and caloric intake, including a bedtime snack, will often lead to a rapid reversal of the troublesome cognitive and confusional lapses and sleep difficulties in these patients (Raskind & Eisdorfer, 1977).

Elderly patients have reduced appetite. They also obtain less sleep, particularly SWS. This generally accepted finding does not consider the possibility that the reduced nighttime sleep is made up by more frequent napping, where SWS predominates. Spiegel (1981) has shown that obese elderly patients have the same sleep stages as normal controls unless they also have related medical problems, in which case REM parameters are reduced. This may have been due to an unreported medication effect. Thus, the general relation between weight loss and reduced sleep may hold in the elderly, even allowing for the high incidence of depression as a confounding variable. It is noted, however, that children increase in weight but decrease total sleep time, a developmental trend that is not consistent with the overall thesis relating weight and sleep changes. Of course, most of the positive findings involve short-term weight changes rather than slower developmental ones.

The literature relating sleep to obesity and weight loss in obese nonpsychiatric patients is quite scanty. Crisp, Stonehill, Fenton, and Fenwick (1973) reported a reduction in total sleep time of over an hour, based on self-reports of five patients whose weight reduced from 100 to 87 kg in four months. One patient was monitored by EEG recordings once a month while reducing from 109 to 76 kg. There was a decrease in total sleep time of about 35 minutes (average). No stage changes other than a decrease in SWS were noted. A pilot report on ten patients, reducing from a mean 172 lb. to about 155 lb. over four months, showed no changes before and after weight loss on three-night recordings in any EEG sleep parameters. Both before and after the weight change the sleep patterns of the ten women were quite typical for age ranges. Although total sleep times were not reported, there were no apparent correlations in their raw data between magnitude of weight loss and REM sleep. However, Adam (1977b) explored the relationship between REM sleep and normal variations in body weight over a 15-week period in 16 nonobese subjects. REM sleep was measured for 20 nights during this period of time after four adaptation nights. The maximum length of sleep was nine hours. A significant correlation of .63 ($p < .01$) was found between total body weight and percentage of REM sleep. Total body weight did not correlate with other sleep parameters. By restricting the data analyzed to the first six hours of sleep, the correlation between total REM sleep and body weight was .65, suggesting that differences in total REM relative to total sleep time did not mediate the results. These correlations were not related to the differences in length of the first three REM cycles in the first half of the night, nor were they related to the variations of age (52 to 67 years of age). This evidence is used by Adam to support her hypothesis that body weight and metabolic rates during sleep are also highly correlated. The results imply that sleep has some function in the restoration of bodily processes. In an apparent continuation study (Adam, 1977a), the difference between the stable, average weight over several months was subtracted from statistical ideal body weight. The periodicity of the REM/non-REM cycle (averaging 90 minutes in healthy adults) was correlated .56 ($p < .03$) with the deviation from ideal body weight, further suggesting that there may be an association between brain rhythms and body weight regulation. These highly speculative studies are in need of replication and extension.

Weight Change, Sleep Disturbance, and REM Sleep

Whatever weight changes contribute to disturbances in sleep, it appears that the disturbances are primarily related to the second half of the night. To the extent that REM occurs late in the typical night, and each successive REM period gets longer (by the end of eight hours of sleep, REM periods may last over 30 minutes, compared to less than five minutes often observed in the first REM period), diminution in total sleep time will almost invariably be associated with a reduction in total REM time. Similarly, an increase in sleep time, particularly if it is continuous sleep time from initial sleep onset, will result in an increase in total REM (but not necessarily the percentage of REM). Increasing REM time at the end of the night may have the same consequences as the debilitating REM rebound effect. There have been no systematic studies to address the possibility that changes in the amount and distribution of REM may play a significant role in the subjective difficulty people report in deliberately maintaining a program of weight loss or weight gain.

Dieting is often associated with amphetamine-based appetite suppressants. Both amphetamines and fenfluramine decrease REM sleep and lead to significant REM rebound effects during withdrawal (Kay et al., 1976; Lewis, Oswald, & Dunleavy, 1971; Oswald, Jones, & Mannerheim, 1968). This was shown by Lewis and co-workers (1971) specifically in obese patients. The subjective effects of the REM rebound may well be instrumental in the difficulties experienced in maintaining an adequate weight-loss program. Weight loss leads to disturbed sleep. The hunger-suppression medications also lead to sleep difficulties, which are accentuated by REM rebound effects during attempts to eliminate medications, or even if the dieter forgets to take them. Thus, subjective effects of sleep dissatisfaction and fatigue increase whenever the medication is withheld, and the dysphoric mood may well be "resolved" by a return to excessive food intake.

The correlation between weight change and changes in sleep patterns may not be a direct causal one. Marked changes in sleep patterns are typically associated with depression. Depressed patients may either increase or decrease sleep with consequent disruptions of sleep stages, particularly fragmentation of REM sleep and a diminution of SWS. Bipolar patients tend to decrease total sleep time, particularly in the early morning during manic episodes. Unipolar patients are as likely to increase as they are to decrease sleep. Thus, the association between weight change and sleep disorders may certainly be mediated through the onset of, or changes in, the course of depressive illness. Crisp and Stonehill (1976) attempted to separate out the relative contributions of depression and weight change in determining sleep loss. They concluded that the association could be shown even in the absence of clinical depression, although the correlation was a very low one.

In summary then, changes in weight are correlated with quality of sleep, probably even when other confounding factors are taken into account. The extent of the relationship and the mechanisms involved require further investigation. The association between weight and sleep can be observed more directly by considering special extreme cases in weight control.

Sleep and Weight Change in Anorexia Nervosa

Crisp and his colleagues have conducted extensive investigations of weight change in the most extreme form of weight loss: anorexia nervosa. In the first of several studies (Crisp & Stonehill, 1971), ten female patients (aged 22 ± 4 years) were studied for eight to 11 weeks during treatment involving restoration to a matched mean population weight for the patients' height. The program included a combination of bed rest, an average of 600 mg of chlorpromazine per day (which would induce sleepiness), a 3,000 calorie balanced diet, and psychotherapy. As the mean group weight increased significantly from 39.9 kg to 54.4 kg ($p < .001$), the self-reported duration of sleep increased from about six and a half to seven and a half hours ($p < .01$), sleep onset time diminished from 67 to 38 minutes ($p < .10$), and a reduction in total time awake during the night fell from 127 minutes to 77 minutes ($p < .02$). These changes were accompanied by more than a 50 percent reduction ($p < .05$) in mean all-night motility scores: both when averages of a three-night period pre- and post-treatment were compared, and when observed on an hour-by-hour basis through the night. The correlation between the amount of weight increase and total sleep time was .56 ($p < .10$); between the change in time of awakening in the morning and weight gain, .89 ($p < .001$). However, sleep-onset time was not correlated with weight change.

In a later study (Crisp, Stonehill, & Fenton, 1971), EEG all-night sleep records were collected for five patients seen ten to 14 days after admission and at the end of treatment. The EEG results compare favorably with the results obtained from the original self-report study. Total hours of sleep increased significantly ($p < .05$) from 6.3 to 7 hours. There were significant pre- to post-treatment increases in SWS ($p < .005$) and REM ($p < .05$) and decreases ($p < .05$) in awakening time through the night. One of the five patients did not change weight. She showed virtually identical sleep-stage patterns before and after treatment.

Lacey, Crisp, Kalucy, Hartmann, and Chen (1975) confirmed the insomnia and early morning awakenings in another ten similar patients. They also confirmed the improvements in total, SWS, and REM sleep as weight recovered to target levels (mean total weight gain was 15 to 25 kg). The increases in sleep occurred particularly over the latter stages of weight gain ($p < .025$). The first half of the weight gain was accompanied by an increase in sleep time of only four minutes, but the change in total sleep time during the second half of the weight gain was from 394 to 441 minutes. The increase in SWS was 58 minutes before a level of 15 percent below target weight was reached, and 113 minutes during the final 15 percent of weight gain. The period of maximum SWS was during the latter part of the weight gain process. At the same time, REM sleep increased over the total time from 99 minutes on admission to 109 minutes at 15 percent below target weight to 139 minutes at full target weight. The overall change in REM sleep ($p < .001$) was about 40 percent. This is not merely a reflection of the longer total sleep period and the consequent increase in REM sleep that would be expected in the second half of the night. When an adjustment was made for length of sleep, the total increase in REM was still about 27 percent. These changes are consistent with data from Phillips, Chen, Crisp, Koval, McGuinness, Kalucy, Kalucy, and Lacey (1975), who found that in normals, high-carbohydrate diets were associated with an increase in REM sleep.

Normal and abnormal EEGs were evaluated in a sample of 55 anorexia patients (six males) in a study by Neil, Merikangas, Foster, Merikangas, Spiker, and Kupfer (1980). While those anorectics with normal EEGs had reasonably normal sleep, those with abnormal waking EEGs had significantly less REM sleep ($p < .01$). Those with EEG abnormalities were more likely to have periods of bulimia.

Although the mechanisms involved are not clear, studies have shown that gonadotropin, steroid, and thyroid abnormalities all return to normal after normalization of body weight in anorectic patients (Boyar, 1978; Crisp & Stonehill, 1976). Whether these abnormalities themselves are a result of malnutrition rather than of primary hypothalamic disturbances is quite controversial.

In summary, the relationship between weight loss and disturbed, diminished sleep is clearly demonstrated in anorexia nervosa patients. It should be noted, however, that depression and anorexia are closely related, and it is possible that the sleep changes relate to changes in depression rather than weight increase. The work of Crisp and his colleagues has documented that, both subjectively and in terms of EEG evidence, anorexia patients sleep poorly with low total sleep time, diminished REM activity, and fragmented and unsatisfying sleep. Improvement in sleep pattern and a return of the integrity of the sleep record accompanies increases in weight during the treatment program of anorectic patients. They sleep best at the time of optimal weight. Sleep changes seem to provide an accurate barometer of clinical progress in these patients. Whether there is a purely nutritional basis to the recovery of sleep or whether there is some other mediating mechanism is not clear.

Obesity and Excessive Daytime Sleepiness

Excessive daytime sleepiness (EDS, lengthy but unsatisfying nighttime sleep, reports of being excessively tired, fatigued, or without energy, frequent daytime catnaps, naps, and sleep attacks) is a common, and often misdiagnosed, medical disorder. Patients often report to sleep clinics with EDS symptoms that have been prevalent for many years. Medical conditions such as hypoglycemia, hypothyroidism, encephalitis, and some brain tumors produce EDS. However, these are relatively rare, particularly in patients with symptoms that have lasted several years. Another group of patients with EDS (frequency unknown) are depressed, have food allergies, or may have recently experienced sudden weight gain. Most complaints of severe EDS are from patients with either narcolepsy or one of several types of sleep apnea. Many of these patients will have a related weight disturbance, usually obesity. Both narcolepsy and sleep apnea are serious and debilitating, and they have been considered extensively in the sleep literature in recent years, probably out of proportion to their incidence as disease entities.

In narcolepsy, sudden attacks of sleep (one to 15 minutes) occur at totally inappropriate times (e.g., while driving, while eating, or during laughter or anger). It may be accompanied by any or all of sleep paralysis, cataplexy, and hypnagogic hallucinations and is difficult to treat. Narcolepsy intrigues sleep researchers because it is the only condition known in which REM occurs at sleep onset (see reviews in Weitzman, 1976). There is a growing recognition of the complex interactions between narcolepsy, a higher than chance incidence of obesity and/or sudden weight gain at the onset of symptoms, and specific food allergies. Indeed, specific foods often trigger the narcoleptic attacks.

The sleep apneas involve serious and debilitating medical problems that have been recognized only in recent years (Gastaut, Tassinari, & Duron, 1965; Sullivan, Henderson-Smart, & Read, 1980). In this disease, patients literally stop breathing at repeated intervals during the night. Following cessation of breathing, for ten seconds or more, sleep lightens to a point where breathing resumes. Patients are often not aware of these sleep apnea spells even though they may occur, accompanied by transient awakenings, over 100 times each night. Presumably, the excessive daytime sleepiness is an attempt to make up for the frequent awakenings during the apnea attacks, and the resultant chronic loss of sleep.

Two pure types of apneas are recognized, though many patients have a mixed type. Central apnea is defined by the total absence of any respiratory effort. The upper airway seems open, but the diaphragm stops moving. Central apnea is rarely associated with obesity. Upper-airway apnea involves a temporary collapse of the airway passages. Respiratory efforts persist but no air is exchanged. Upper-airway apnea is often associated with obesity. In a series of 30 patients studied intensively by Guilleminault and Dement (1978), 63 percent were at least 15 percent overweight. Apnea is a debilitating disease resulting in intellectual, cognitive, and personality impairment, automatic behavior and abnormal outbursts, hypertension, cardiovascular disease, and other disturbances. Apnea is easily differentially diagnosed from narcolepsy because of the cycle of loud snoring–intermittent silence during the airway obstruction.

Attacks are often stimulated by a particular sleep position, often lying on the back. Therapy may consist of attempts to control the person's sleep position. This may involve a sleeping partner, mechanical devices such as a marble sewed in the back of pajamas, or special constraints. In more extreme cases, radical treatments such as surgical removal of excessive fat deposits, permanent tracheostomy, or, in the extremely obese, bypass surgery may be required. In obese patients with EDS and sleep apnea, dieting, even with weight loss of up to 30 kg, is of mixed and limited success. In children, removal of the tonsils and adenoids usually eliminates the symptoms. When EDS is accompanied by massive obesity, it is usually referred to as the "Pickwickian syndrome," after the well-known Dickens character. Roth (1978) is one of the few clinicians who finds that weight loss of 15 to 20 kg in Pickwickian patients leads to improvement in EDS. He recommends this weight loss be accompanied by small doses of central stimulants such as methylphenidate. These medications should be withdrawn with extreme caution, during hospitalization, because of the REM rebound-induced irregular respiration.

The so-called Klein–Levin syndrome is also widely discussed but extremely rare. Periods of excessive sleepiness are coupled with increased appetites for food and sex accompanied by confusion and retrograde amnesia for waking periods. Polyphagia and bulimia can lead to dramatic weight swings (Critchley, 1962). Food ingestion is based more on its availability than on hunger. Klein–Levin syndrome is usually found in adolescent males, often following febrile illness. Obesity follows rather than precedes initial onset, and the prognosis is good. Crisp and Stonehill (1976) point to the similarity between what has been considered exclusively a male disease (Klein–Levin) and what has been exclusively a female disease (anorexia). During weight gain in anorectic females, bouts of overeating accompanied by confusional states are often encountered. Bouts of bulimia are usually terminated by self-induced vomiting or sleep. They argue that neither disease is sex-limited.

In summary, the most commonly recognized psychiatric syndromes associated with EDS—narcolepsy, sleep apnea, Pickwickian and Klein–Levin syndromes—are clearly associated to varying degrees with obesity. In extreme form, EDS gives strong support to Crisp's hypothesis that excessive weight and excessive sleep are related. However, evidence that obesity is a causal or mediating factor in sleep apnea EDS, except in an almost mechanical sense, is lacking.

Nutrition and Sleep

While the work of Crisp has shown an apparent clear-cut relationship between sudden weight loss and disturbed sleep, on the one hand, and weight gain and increased restful sleep, on the other, the mechanisms involved are not in fact clear. The hypothesis developed by Crisp is that this is due to the nutritional status of the individual. However, there has been very little work done linking specific nutritional variables and sleep parameters. This review will focus on L-tryptophan (a naturally occurring amino acid precursor of serotonin), beverages (other than alcohol), bedtime snacks, and food allergies.

L-Tryptophan and Sleep

Most of us are familiar with the postprandial drowsiness commonly experienced after the lunchtime meal. This well-known phenomenon may not be a result of caloric intake, but may be related to the ingestion of L-tryptophan, which is found in many foods. L-Tryptophan is abundant in such natural sources as milk, cereal, meat, fish, and nuts. Normal diets result in an intake of L-tryptophan of .5 to 2 gm per day. It has recently been proposed as a safe and effective sleep-inducing medication.

L-Tryptophan is an essential amino acid and is the natural physiological precursor of serotonin. Serotonin is involved in the modulation of SWS and may well be implicated in the triggering of REM sleep. A number of studies investigating the effects of L-tryptophan on sleep patterns have produced confusing results. Several excellent reviews of this literature now exist (Cole, Hartmann, & Brigham, 1980; Hartmann, 1978; Wyatt & Gillin, 1976), and some general, but still tentative conclusions can be drawn based on over a dozen, mostly well-controlled blind studies.

1. At dosages below 1 gm (equivalent to about .5 kg meat dish), its effect on sleep is unclear (Hartmann, Cravens, & List, 1974; Hartmann & Spinweber, 1979; Oswald, Berger, Evans, & Thacore, 1964).

2. At moderate doses of 1 gm and above, reasonably consistent dose–response curves are obtained, indicating that L-tryptophan reduces sleep-onset latency and nighttime awakenings and increases total sleep time and SWS (Hartmann, 1978; Hartmann et al., 1974).

3. The detection of sleep-onset effects is in part a function of baseline sleep-onset latencies. For normal sleepers, particularly those who fall asleep in ten minutes or less, L-tryptophan, not surprisingly, has little or no effect on sleep onset. For mild (onset more than 20 minutes) and moderate insomnia, the effects on onset are quite significant (Cole et al., 1980). Patients with serious insomnia (typical onset latencies greater than an hour) have not been studied.

4. There is some evidence that initial effects of L-tryptophan on sleep do not appear until after ten days to a month of repeated same-dose administration.

5. Doses between 1 and 7 gm, during daytime or evening periods, induce subjective sleepiness, as measured on the Stanford Sleepiness Scale (Hoddes, Zarcone, Smythe, Phillips, & Dement, 1973).

6. Large doses (15 gm) may increase REM sleep (Griffiths, Lester, Coulter, & Williams, 1972). This challenging study requires replication.

7. At least three studies suggest that L-tryptophan has relatively little effect in improving sleep in depressed patients. This is a disappointing result and requires further investigation, as large doses of L-tryptophan may or may not have antidepressant effects (Cole et al., 1980; Hartmann, 1978). Some positive

effects of L-tryptophan on depression have been found in combination with MAO inhibitors and in hypomania. This area of research is difficult to evaluate.

Because of the widespread publicity given to the L-tryptophan studies, investigations of the possible mechanisms and limiting factors have recently been conducted.

Wyatt, Engleman, Kupfer, Fram, Sjoerdsma, and Snyder (1970) reported that when L-tryptophan was given in moderate doses to three patients in whom synthesis of serotonin was partially blocked by para-chlorophenylalanine (PCPA), the PCPA pretreatment decreased REM but did not reduce the tryptophan's sedative effects. SWS was increased, as expected, following PCPA blockade. Thus, whether the action of L-tryptophan on sleep involves serotonin levels is questionable—a finding that is not entirely surprising given that only a small amount of the body's tryptophan is converted to serotonin. Tryptophan is metabolized to tryptamine and kynurenine as well as serotonin. Wyatt and Gillin (1976) summarize preliminary evidence suggesting that the effects of L-tryptophan on sleep are not mediated through tryptamine (MAO inhibitors do not block the sedative effects of tryptophan) and kynurenine (which has no specific effects on sleep, either alone or through its derivative, nicotinamide acid).

Both tryptophan and tyrosine that had been labeled by radioactive carbon were administered to normal volunteers (Rodden, Sinhas, Dement, Berchas, Zarcone, MacLeury, & DeGrazia, 1973). There were no differences between waking and sleeping rates of metabolism for tyrosine, but there was a three-fold slowing of the excretion of tryptophan during sleep.

Most (up to 90 percent) of total plasma tryptophan is bound to albumin; there is a smaller free tryptophan fraction (10 to 20 percent). It is not free plasma tryptophan but rather the ratio of free tryptophan to neutral amino acids that is related to total brain serotonin levels. Neither free nor bound tryptophan showed any direct temporal relationship to sleep stages (Chen, Kalucy, Hartmann, Lacey, Crisp, Bailey, Eccleston, & Coppen, 1974). However, the mean free tryptophan levels for the whole night were positively correlated with total percentage of REM sleep, but negatively correlated with percentage of SWS. The reverse was found for bound plasma tryptophan; levels were related positively to SWS and negatively to REM sleep.

It seems clear that moderate ingestion of L-tryptophan may have beneficial effects on some sleep parameters, at least over a short period, and there are only relatively mild side effects (euphoria on arousal, nausea) for even large doses. Unfortunately, the biochemical picture is much more complex than the total ingestion of this natural substance would suggest. L-Tryptophan is an amino acid precursor of serotonin: production of serotonin depends on the availability of tryptophan, which crosses the blood–brain barrier on a transport protein. There are six major competing amino acids for the same transport protein, and tryptophan has the lowest affinity of any of the group. Thus, increased amounts of free (or total) tryptophan do not necessarily enter the brain unless blood concentrations of tryptophan are increased relative to the competing concentration of the other amino acids (Fernstrom & Wurtman, 1974). In addition, high-carbohydrate feedings increase total plasma tryptophan and consequently brain tryptophan and serotonin levels. However, with balanced diets and meals supplemented with protein, the availability of brain tryptophan, relative to larger amounts of the other neutral amino acids, may decrease (Cole et al., 1980; Hartmann, Crisp, Evans, Gaitonde, & Kirkwood, 1979).

Serotonergic mechanisms are not only implicated in the control of sleep onset (or possibly the transition from SWS to other stages of sleep), but may also be involved in depression. It has already been pointed out that SWS is decreased in depression and increases during recovery. The association between eating and weight disorders on the one hand, and sleep mechanisms on the other, is consistently confounded with the frequent occurrence of depressive symptomatology in the patients upon whom data are available. L-Tryptophan has been used in large doses as a naturally occurring treatment of depression, again with mixed clinical results. All of the biochemical questions relevant to the evaluation of L-tryptophan in sleep are equally relevant to its use in depression. Existing studies are not definitive and suffer from a number of methodological difficulties (see Cole et al., 1980, for the most comprehensive review to date). Unless attempts are made to change the balance of competing amino acids, particularly relative to tyrosine, the evidence suggesting that tryptophan directly affects depression is indeed controversial. It is tempting to suggest a trial with tryptophan in the treatment of patients with a sleep disorder (sleep-onset or sleep-maintenance insomnia) who are depressed (particularly bipolar illness), combined with a high-carbohydrate, low-protein, easy-to-digest diet. The common error will likely be to overtreat the sleep and weight problems while undertreating the depression, as is so often the case when the sedative effects of tricyclic antidepressants at low dosages are misinterpreted as appropriate clinical dosages for the treatment of the depression itself. As with tricyclics, there is the danger that treatment may be curtailed before levels are sufficient to serve as an antidepressant even though symptomatic treatment may well occur in terms of both the improvement in sleep and possible resurgence of appetite.

While it is currently difficult to predict the level of L-tryptophan adequate to reduce sleep onset and improve the quality of sleep, there is no question that there are metabolic processes involved in the regulation of eating that interact with tryptophan and its availability to the brain. These mechanisms are not yet well understood and are worthy of further study, particularly as tryptophan may be a relatively safe substance, without serious side effects. Its careful use may help regulate at least the sleep process, if not the depression process, in those patients where sleep and weight disorders are linked by some unknown mechanisms.

Beverages and Bedtime Snacks

A number of studies have documented the beneficial effects of either hot milk or proprietary beverages, such as Horlicks or Ovaltine, that consist of grain-derived drinks mixed with (warm) milk. It is common folklore that such beverages are natural aids to sleep. Indeed, over 40 years ago, Laird and Drexel (1934) found that a bedtime snack of cornflakes and milk, a relatively easily digested snack, compared to a specially prepared less easily digested meal led to sleep accompanied by fewer body movements, implying improved, less disturbed sleep. The motility change in the cereal group was about 16 percent. Kleitman and co-workers (1937) showed that sleep was more restless after a malted milk drink than after other forms of bedtime nourishment, including hot and cold milk and hot and cold water. They found 14 gm, but not 8 gm, of Ovaltine, in either hot or cold milk or water, significantly decreased motility during sleep and tended to reduce sleep-onset latency, as well as the subjective satisfaction with sleep on awakening. Giddings (1934) also found that warm milk at bedtime, but not cold milk or water, decreased motility in approximately half of the 12 children he studied. Using time-lapse cinematography, Southwell, Evans, and Hunt (1972) found that a malted milk beverage (Horlicks) was associated with a reduced number of body movements in medical students during sleep. The reduction of movement with Horlicks compared to hot milk or a no-drink control was significant ($p < .02$). Because motility is not a good indicator of sleep parameters, and because these studies were not blind, the results are, at best, suggestive.

Brezinova and Oswald (1972) repeated these studies, monitoring sleep by EEG methods in a group of ten young adults and an older group of eight adults (mean age of 55 years). They compared a 32-gm Horlicks and 250-ml hot milk drink with a yellow capsule; the findings of Southwell and colleagues (1972) were replicated. In both groups a significant reduction in body movement, as measured by EEG sleep criteria, occurred ($p < .02$), particularly late in the night. The effect on the elderly group was even more dramatic, particularly late at night. The length of sleep increased significantly ($p < .05$) and the number of nighttime awakenings decreased ($p < .02$). There were no specific effects on stages of sleep.

The best of these studies was recently reported by Adam (1980) in which 16 volunteers (aged 52 to 67) were monitored by EEG criteria under blind randomized conditions: (1) inert capsule; (2) 284 ml milk; (3) 32 gm of Horlicks and 284 ml milk; and (4) a flavored drink designed to be nutritionally equivalent (energy, protein, carbohydrate, and fat) to the malted barley and wheat based Horlicks. She found that the cereal beverage led to less wakefulness and more drowsiness during the first six hours of sleep. The effects were small unless habitual nutritional intake of the subjects prior to bedtime was considered. The more a person usually ate before bedtime, the greater the sleep impairment following the nutritionally inert capsule compared to milk and Horlicks; but the less the subject usually ate before bedtime, the less the advantage for milk and Horlicks in facilitating restful sleep. There were no differences for bedtime eaters or non-bedtime eaters favoring the Horlicks or milk groups in terms of sleep onset and SWS or REM sleep periods. The correlation between typical bedtime food consumption and the improvement in restful sleep time induced by Horlicks was .68 ($p < .01$). This study serves to warn that studies in this area are fraught with difficulty and that nutritional history during the 24-hour period may be one of the potent variables affecting results.

These studies, though limited, do show some advantage to cereal and cereal-based beverages before bedtime in terms of decreasing nighttime wakefulness and awakenings and, less clearly, on sleep-onset speed. The mechanisms are not clear. The favorite hypothesis is that milk and the cereal-based drinks contain l-tryptophan: tryptophan may have some benefit in reducing sleep-onset latency, decreasing restlessness, and increasing sleep satisfaction.

The tryptophan hypothesis is by no means clear-cut, and other mechanisms could be implicated. Warm milk is of course a well-known sleep-inducing substance in the newborn infant, and the possibility that there is some learned expectational factor involved in these studies must be considered. Lust (1921, cited by Kleitman, 1963) found that intramuscular injections of 2 ml of milk produced restful rapid onset sleep in a sleepless child following an attack of encephalitis. Interestingly, the child's body temperature was raised from 37.3 to 37.8°C by the injections of milk. While sleep usually occurs when temperature is dropping (Dinges et al., 1980), increases in core temperature induce REM sleep.

Pfeiffer (1979) points out that milk contains both calcium and magnesium, and he cites unsupported clinical data suggesting that both of these are beneficial in reducing sleep onset time. Both are slightly increased in cats' brains during sleep (Kleitman, 1963), and it has been shown that calcium injected into cats' brains induces immediate sleep. Pavlinac and colleagues (1978) have shown in preliminary studies that plasma calcium and magnesium both showed spectral analysis peaks during sleep. Plasma calcium and magnesium concentrations are in phase with REM sleep. Calcium–REM relationships were confirmed by Kripke and associates (1978). Other data suggest that SWS is related to a variety of metabolic and anabolic processes (e.g., glucose metabolism; Macho & Sinha, 1980). A number of studies have shown that growth hormone release and a thyroid-releasing hormone are both particularly active during SWS (Dunleavy, Oswald, Brown, & Strong, 1974; Wyatt & Gillin, 1976). Adam and Oswald (1977a,b) have speculated and Rojas-Ramirez and co-workers (1976) have provided animal data that suggest that REM sleep is related to increased protein metabolism. Drucker-Colin (1981) has shown that protein levels of the extracellular fluid peak cyclically corresponding to periods in which REM sleep occupies the largest percentage of time. Sleep deprivation eliminates this cyclic protein release. Not only are protein levels higher during REM than during awakening, but REM sleep perfusates contain two proteins not present in awake perfusates or serum samples. Protein-synthesis inhibitors reduce REM time, or at least REM-period frequency. In all-night polygraph studies of four children (ages six to nine years) with a history of malnutrition, REM sleep was chronically reduced by 53 percent of levels in normal control children.

Although the protein synthesis hypothesis fares favorably with the tryptophan hypothesis, it does not account for the cereal beverage data. Other nutritional components may be implicated in these studies. Phillips and colleagues (1975) showed that in similar isocaloric diets, high versus low carbohydrate levels (with protein levels equated) significantly decreased SWS (from 25.4 percent, normal, to 21.5 percent, high carbohydrate) but increased REM sleep (from 23.1 percent on normal diet to 30.1 percent and 26.9 percent on high versus low carbohydrate). This unbalanced non-blind study requires replication. It is one of the few studies showing non-rebound-related increases in

REM sleep. In a related study, Lacey and associates (1975) showed that the standard high-carbohydrate treatment diet of ten anorexia patients also increased REM sleep from 26.0 percent to 33.0 percent ($p <$ .005) of total sleep time. About two-thirds of this REM increase occurred after the time when the patients had reached within 15 percent of their target weight, the time when major endocrine and metabolic changes take place. Total sleep time increased in these ten patients by about 41 minutes, most of which would be spent in REM sleep (at the end of the sleep period when the anorexia patients have maximal sleep disturbance). The increase in sleep time is not sufficient to account for the total increase in REM (of 41 minutes). In the three studies reviewed, increased carbohydrate intake was accompanied by increased fat intake (but not necessarily protein), and the relative contribution of carbohydrate/fat ratios is unknown.

In another isocaloric diet-controlled study, Lacey, Stanley, Hartmann, Koval, and Crisp (1978) compared nighttime infusion of saline, glucose, and amino acid in nine subjects (mean age of 21.2) over four nights maintained on a controlled diet. The amino acid was delivered by aminosol, a dialyzed hydrolysate of casein. They found that SWS was significantly ($p <$ .01) increased (to 31.6 percent) in the aminosol group compared to glucose (29 percent) and saline (24 percent, a typical SWS baseline level) even though the total sleep time was nonsignificantly shorter for the aminosol nights compared to the others. Aminosol also slightly increased sleep-onset latency and REM time ($p <$ .002). These data are consistent with a hypothesized increase in anabolic activity in SWS. It is worth noting that chemical manipulations do not typically increase SWS in normal adults (Hartmann, 1978), though they do in depressed insomnia patients who have markedly reduced SWS baselines.

To summarize, there is preliminary evidence that specific nutrients may affect sleep onset, percent REM and SWS stages, and the restfulness of and subjective satisfaction with sleep. The available findings are not, in general, derived from well-controlled studies. L-Tryptophan, protein synthesis, carbohydrate/fat ratios, glucose metabolism, and other factors have been implicated. This area is "hungry" for further research.

Caffeine

It is well known that many people suffer from sleep-onset insomnia following the ingestion of caffeine before retiring. A number of studies has documented this effect.

Brezinova (1974) examined the effects of 300 mg of caffeine in six healthy middle-aged adults compared to decaffeinated coffee and a no-drug condition. This carefully replicated balanced-order design showed that caffeine decreased total sleep and increased sleep-onset latency, nocturnal wakefulness, and number of nighttime awakenings and post-sleep drowsiness. REM sleep and SWS were decreased, but probably only proportionally to the decrease in total sleep time. Older subjects had more sleep disturbance after caffeine than younger subjects in the sample.

These results have been replicated by Karacan, Thornby, Booth, Okawa, Salis, Anch, and Williams (1975). They found dose-related decreases in total sleep time, increases in sleep-onset latency and transient awakenings ($N = 18$ healthy young males).

Not all individuals seem to be seriously affected by the ingestion of caffeine close to bedtime. There are also popular misconceptions about the quantity of caffeine in different beverages. For example, caffeine content of percolated coffee is not very different from instant coffee or tea (though its effects may be modulated by interactions with tannin and other chemicals in the latter). Caffeine is also present in similar quantities in soft drinks, particularly cola varieties. The cola drinks are especially a problem in terms of sleep-onset difficulty because of the combined stimulant effects of caffeine and the significant incidence of allergic reaction to cola drinks, particularly in children.

In psychiatric patients, the implications of caffeine use are often not recognized. Hospitalized psychotic patients consume high levels of caffeine (and nicotine) if it is available. One study suggests caffeine may pose special problems for unipolar depressed patients who sometimes use it for its temporary and possibly illusory antidepressant (stimulant) effects (Neil, Himmelhoch, Mallinger, Mallinger, & Hanin, 1978). Fighting the hypersomnic episodes with caffeine, accentuated by the possible interaction between caffeine and standard pharmacological therapy, may prolong illness in depressed patients. Caffeine and tricyclic medications might well have antagonistic effects on sleep cycles. Neil and co-workers (1978) reported that withdrawal of caffeine, particularly in unipolar depressed patients, produced more rapid therapeutic change. This has not been confirmed yet in well-designed double-blind studies.

Lutz (1978) has recently shown that caffeine was an important etiological factor in 62 patients with "restless legs" syndrome. This is a troublesome syndrome associated with sleep involving an unpleasant creeping sensation in the lower legs, typically between the knee and ankle, resulting in awakening with an irresistable need to move the limbs. It is typically accompanied by severe insomnia. Impressive clinical material is presented showing the syndrome may be alleviated by abstinence from all beverages and medications (including some pain-relieving drugs) containing caffeine.

Food and Beverage Allergies and Sleep Disorders

Perhaps the most neglected area in evaluating the relationship between eating, weight modulation, and sleep disturbances relates to specific food allergies. Allergists (e.g., Bray, 1931) have long realized that excessive fatigue, disturbed sleep, and hypersomnia are common side effects of food allergies. Yet most reviews of sleep disorders typically assert that over 85 percent of patients with hypersomnia involve narcolepsy or sleep apnea; the remainder are likely to involve hypothyroidism or other rare medical conditions.

The incidence of food allergy as a determinant of sleep disorders has been studied carefully only in a few investigations. As an example, Bell, Guilleminault, and Dement (1978) reported a case study of a moderately obese 39-year-old patient who had a highly selective IgA deficiency and dysomnia, as well as a long history of undiagnosed psychiatric illness. The psychiatric disturbance and excessive daytime sleepiness were successfully treated by eliminating a large number of allergenic substances, many of which were food related. However, following the remission of psychiatric symptoms, IgA levels did not return to normal limits. Sugerman, Southern, and Rizvi (1980) reviewed several studies reporting increased incidences of food allergies in psychiatric patients, particularly schizophrenics and alcoholics, and reported elevated IgE levels in schizophrenics, alcoholics, and depressed consecutive patient admissions, compared to a control group. None of the studies reviewed referred to sleep difficulties.

Breneman (1978) reviewed several surveys in which 83 to 90 percent of children with diagnosed food allergies also had primary nocturnal enuresis. Frequently, elimination of offending foods from the diet led to immediate symptom remission. In these studies, milk was found to be the primary allergen in about 60 percent of the allergic children (and even in about 10 percent of newborn infants). Eggs, citrus fruits, corn, wheat, tomato, and chocolate were implicated in more than 10 percent of the allergenic, enuretic children. In a large sample (Campbell, 1973) of 654 carefully evaluated consecutive adult patients in an allergy clinic, about 75 percent had significant food allergies. Insomnia was reported in 19 percent, and periods of excessive tiredness that were unrelieved by sleep were reported by 38 percent of these patients. Like the enuretic children, chocolate (37 percent), milk (35 percent), nuts (19 percent), coffee (19 percent), pork (19 percent), tomatoes (19 percent), citrus fruits (18 percent), wheat (18 percent), shellfish (10 percent), and eggs (10 percent) were foods producing the most frequent positive allergy reactions in those with insomnia or hypersomnia.

There are reports that excessive intake of food and/or food allergies can serve as a trigger stimulus for the onset of narcoleptic sleep attacks (Bell, Hawley, Guilleminault, & Dement, 1976). Randolph (1979) suggested that alcohol addiction may be derived from masked allergies to wheat, barley, corn, and other grains. However, there was no support for this hypothesis in the pilot study by Sugerman and colleagues (1980).

Similarly, food allergies and additives have been controversially linked to hyperactivity over recent years. Unfortunately, the relationship between food allergens, hyperactivity, and EEG-documented sleep disturbances in hyperactive children has not been studied systematically.

The frequency of allergy to coffee (and to a lesser extent, tea) suggests a possible explanation for the unusually broad individual differences in pre-sleep tolerance of coffee and caffeine-based drinks. There is also no documentation available of the pediatricians' clinical observations linking sleep difficulties, and especially early night enuresis, in children ingesting significant quantities of cola-type drinks. Presumably, caffeine is the mediating substance. There are undocumented clinical impressions that in children with serious sleep disorders (enuresis, disturbed sleep, excessive daytime sleepiness), controlled diet manipulation and allergen testing, particularly of the liquids and foods mentioned, should be an early therapeutic consideration.

It was recently reported (Marks, 1980) that bruxism (nocturnal toothgrinding) is specifically associated with allergies. There is a threefold increase in the incidence of nocturnal bruxism in children with specific allergies (primarily food related) compared to nonallergic children. Marks carefully documented a strong link between the allergic edema of mucosal membrane of the tympanic cavity and edema induced by intermittent blockage of the eustachian tube.

Preliminary reports have indicated that postprandial drowsiness, experienced particularly after the noontime meal, may be more pronounced following the ingestion of certain foods (Bell, Blair, Owens,

Guilleminault, & Dement, 1976). These studies have shown that different foods have different effects on the pre-post meal ratings of the Stanford Sleepiness Scale (Hoddes et al., 1973). Foods with high L-tryptophan levels are prominent in the list of sleepiness-inducing substances. This was subsequently confirmed (Bell, Rosekind, Hargrave, Guilleminault, & Dement, 1977) by feeding 12 normal volunteer students one of four isovolumic meals. Postlunchtime sleepiness was greatest in the tryptophan feedings, followed by, in descending order, corn oil, dextrose, and water-control feeding groups.

It should be noted that several of the major allergenic foods are typically foods also high in L-tryptophan and other competing amino acids that have been implicated in facilitating sleep and drowsiness. This suggests an as yet untested hypothesis that may help to account for some of the confusing data on L-tryptophan and improved sleep. It is possible that L-tryptophan facilitates sleep onset and prolonged restful sleep in most individuals, but its beneficial effects may interact with or be canceled by specific food allergies.

Conclusion

A number of tentative conclusions, each requiring further research, can be drawn about the relationship between eating, weight disorders, and sleep.

Sudden changes in weight are associated with corresponding changes in sleep patterns. Weight loss is associated with disturbances in sleep and restless and truncated sleep, resulting in a reduction in REM time. The negative effects of REM rebound may well contribute to the difficulty many people have in maintaining a weight-loss program. Weight gain is associated with increases in total sleep time, SWS and REM sleep, and mild hypersomnia. The mediating role of depression in these changes in weight and sleep must always be suspected, but it is not clear what causal mechanisms are responsible.

Obese patients suffering from severe excessive daytime sleepiness without evidence of increasing weight should be evaluated for either narcolepsy or, more likely, sleep apnea.

Hypersomnia can occasionally be caused by specific food allergies. Food allergies should be considered seriously when children report sleep difficulties. Food allergies may also often be implicated in such sleep-related disorders as enuresis, particularly if it occurs in the first half of the night, and bruxism.

The regulation of diet and bedtime eating may be beneficial to people suffering from insomnia, particularly sleep-onset insomnia. A bedtime snack, particularly if it consists of nonallergenic foods or beverages, may be beneficial to sleep onset and subjectively satisfying sleep. Helpful snacks include warm milk and cereal, grain-based beverages other than alcohol, or snacks including milk, nuts, and meat, which are high in the natural amino acid precursor of serotonin, L-tryptophan. L-Tryptophan shows considerable promise as a safe, naturally occurring sleeping "medication," though its regulation in terms of carbohydrate/protein ratios, competing amino acids, and food allergies complicate its usage. Coffee, tea, and cola drinks should be avoided by those adults and children who have sleep-onset difficulties.

While some of the findings discussed have not been subject to definitive, well-controlled studies, it is clear that they are important in understanding the relationship between our two main vegetative functions, sleeping and eating.

References

Adam, K. Percentage REM sleep is correlated with body weight. *Sleep Research*, 1977, *6*, 41. (a)

Adam, K. Sleep cycle duration correlates with percentage deviation from ideal body weight. *Sleep Research*, 1977, *6*, 42. (b)

Adam, K. Dietary habits and sleep after bedtime food drinks. *Sleep*, 1980, *3*, 47–58.

Adam, K., & Oswald, I. Sleep is for tissue restoration. *Journal of the Royal College of Physicians*, 1977, *11*, 376–388. (a)

Adam, K., & Oswald, I. Why sleep is a time of greater net protein synthesis. *Sleep Research*, 1977, *6*, 63. (b)

Aserinsky, E., & Kleitman, N. Regularly occurring periods of eye motility and concomitant phenomena during sleep. *Science*, 1953, *118*, 273–274.

Beck, A. T. *Depression: Clinical, experimental and theoretical aspects.* London: Staples Press, 1967.

Bell, I. R., Blair, S. R., Owens, M., Guilleminault, C., & Dement, W. C. Post-prandial sleepiness after specific foods in normals. *Sleep Research*, 1976, *5*, 41.

Bell, I. R., Guilleminault, C., & Dement, W. C. Hypersomnia, multiple-system symptomatology, and selective IgA deficiency. *Biological Psychiatry*, 1978, *13*, 751–757.

Bell, I. R., Hawley, C. D., Guilleminault, C., & Dement, W. C. Diet and symptom histories in food allergics versus narcoleptics and normals. *Sleep Research*, 1976, *5*, 155.

Bell, I. R., Rosekind, M., Hargrave, V., Guilleminault, C., & Dement, W. C.

Lunchtime sleepiness and nap sleep after specific foods in normals. *Sleep Research,* 1977, *6,* 45.

Boyar, R. M. Endocrine changes in anorexia nervosa. *Medical Clinics of North America,* 1978, *62,* 297–303.

Bray, G. W. Enuresis of allergic origin. *Archives of Disease in Childhood,* 1931, *6,* 251–253.

Breneman, J. C. *Basics of food allergy.* Springfield, Ill.: Charles C Thomas, 1978.

Brezinova, V. Effect of caffeine on sleep: EEG study in late middle age people. *British Journal of Clinical Pharmacology,* 1974, *1,* 203–208.

Brezinova, V., & Oswald, I. Sleep after a bedtime beverage. *British Medical Journal,* 1972, *2,* 431–433.

Campbell, M. B. Neurologic manifestations of allergic disease. *Annals of Allergy,* 1973, *31,* 485–497.

Carney, M. W. P., Roth, M., & Garside, R. F. The diagnosis of depressive syndromes and the prediction of ECT response. *British Journal of Psychiatry,* 1965, *111,* 659–674.

Chen, C. N., Kalucy, R. S., Hartmann, M. K., Lacey, J. H., Crisp, A. H., Bailey, J. E., Eccleston, E. G., & Coppen, A. Plasma tryptophan and sleep. *British Journal of Medicine,* 1974, *4,* 564–566.

Cole, J. O., Hartmann, E., & Brigham, P. L-Trytophan: Clinical studies. In J. O. Cole (Ed.), *Psychopharmacology update.* Lexington, Mass.: The Collamore Press, 1980.

Crisp, A. H., & Stonehill, E. Aspects of the relationship between psychiatric status, sleep, nocturnal motility and nutrition. *Journal of Psychosomatic Research,* 1971, *15,* 501–509.

Crisp, A. H., & Stonehill, E. *Sleep, nutrition and mood.* London: John Wiley & Sons, 1976.

Crisp, A. H., Stonehill, E., & Fenton, G. W. The relationship between sleep, nutrition and mood: A study of patients with anorexia nervosa. *Postgraduate Medical Journal,* 1971, *47,* 207–213.

Crisp, A. H., Stonehill, E., Fenton, G. W., & Fenwick, P. B. C. Sleep patterns in obese patients during weight reduction. *Psychotherapy and Psychosomatics,* 1973, *22,* 159–165.

Critchley, M. Periodic hypersomnia and megaphagia in adolescent males. *Brain,* 1962, *85,* 627–656.

Danguir, J., & Nicolaidis, S. Dependence of sleep on nutrients' availability. *Physiology and Behavior,* 1979, *22,* 735–740.

Dement, W., & Kleitman, N. Cyclic variations in EEG during sleep and their relation to eye movements, body motility, and dreaming. *Electroencephalography and Clinical Neurophysiology,* 1957, *9,* 673–690.

Dinges, D. F., Orne, M. T., Orne, E. C., & Evans, F. J. Voluntary self-control of sleep to facilitate quasi-continuous performance (Report No. 80). Washington, D.C.: U.S. Army Medical Research and Development Command, March, 1980.

Drucker-Colin, R. P. Neuroproteins, brain excitability, and REM sleep. In W. Fishbein (Ed.), *Sleep, dreams, and memory.* New York: Spectrum Publications, 1981.

Dunleavy, D. L. F., Oswald, I., Brown, P., & Strong, J. A. Hyperthyroidism, sleep and growth hormone. *Electroencephalography and Clinical Neurophysiology,* 1974, *36,* 259–263.

Fara, J. W., Rubinstein, E. H., & Sonnenschein, R. R. Visceral and behavioral responses to intraduodenal fat. *Science,* 1969, *166,* 110–111.

Fernstrom, J. D., & Wurtman, R. J. Nutrition and the brain. *Scientific American,* 1974, *230,* 84–91.

Gastaut, H., Tassinari, C. A., & Duron, B. Etude polygraphique des manifestations épisodiques (hypniques et respiratoires), diurnes et nocturnes, du syndrome de Pickwick. *Revue Neurologique,* 1965, *112,* 568–579.

Giddings, G. Child's sleep—effect of certain food and beverages on sleep motility. *American Journal of Public Health,* 1934, *24,* 609–614.

Gold, M. S., Pottash, A. L. C., Davies, R. K., Ryan, N., Sweeney, D. R., & Martin, D. M. Distinguishing unipolar and bipolar depression by thyrotropin release test. *The Lancet,* 1979, *2,* 411–412.

Griffiths, W. J., Lester, B. K., Coulter, J. D., & Williams, H. L. Tryptophan and sleep in young adults. *Psychophysiology,* 1972, *9,* 345–356.

Guilleminault, C., & Dement, W. C. Sleep apnea syndromes and related sleep disorders. In R. L. Williams & I. Karacan (Eds.), *Sleep disorders: Diagnosis and treatment.* New York: John Wiley & Sons, 1978.

Hall, W. H., Orr, W. C., & Stahl, M. Gastric function during sleep. *Sleep Research,* 1976, *5,* 43.

Hartmann, E. *The sleeping pill.* New Haven: Yale University Press, 1978.

Hartmann, E., Cravens, J., & List, S. Hypnotic effects of L-tryptophan. *Archives of General Psychiatry,* 1974, *31,* 394–397.

Hartmann, M. K., Crisp, A. H., Evans, G., Gaitonde, M. K., & Kirkwood, B. R. Short-term effects of CHO, fat, and protein loads on total tryptophan/tyrosine levels in plasma as related to % REM sleep. *Waking and Sleeping,* 1979, *3,* 63.

Hartmann, E., & Spinweber, C. Sleep induced by L-tryptophan: Effects of dosages within the normal dietary intake. *Journal of Nervous and Mental Disorders,* 1979, *167,* 497–499.

Hoddes, E., Zarcone, V., Smythe, H., Phillips, R., & Dement, W. C. Quantification of sleepiness: A new approach. *Psychophysiology,* 1973, *10,* 431–436.

Jacobs, B. L., & McGinty, D. J. Effects of food deprivation on sleep and wakefulness in the rat. *Experimental Neurology,* 1971, *30,* 212–222.

Johnson, L. C. Are stages of sleep related to waking behavior? *American Scientist,* 1973, *61,* 326–338.

Kales, A., & Kales, J. D. Recent findings in the diagnosis and treatment of disturbed sleep. *New England Journal of Medicine,* 1974, *290,* 487.

Karacan, I., Thornby, J. I., Booth, G. H., Okawa, M., Salis, P. J., Anch, A. M., & Williams, R. L. Dose-response effects of coffee on objective (EEG) and subjective measures of sleep. In P. Levin & W. P. Koella (Eds.), *Sleep 1974.* Basel, Switzerland: S. Karger, 1975.

Kay, D. C., Blackburn, A. B., Buckingham, J. A., & Karacan, I. Human pharmacology of sleep. In R. L. Williams & I. Karacan (Eds.), *Pharmacology of sleep*. New York: John Wiley & Sons, 1976.

Kiloh, L. G., & Garside, R. F. The independence of neurotic depression and endogenous depression. *British Journal of Psychiatry*, 1963, *109*, 451–463.

Kleitman, N. *Sleep and wakefulness* (Rev. ed.). Chicago: The University of Chicago Press, 1963.

Kleitman, N., Mullin, F. J., Cooperman, N. R., & Titelbaum, S. *Sleep characteristics*. Chicago: The University of Chicago Press, 1937.

Kripke, D. F., Lavie, P., Parker, D., Huey, L., & Deftos, L. J. Plasma parathyroid hormone and calcium are related to sleep stage cycles. *Journal of Clinical Endocrinology and Metabolism*, 1978, *47*, 1021–1027.

Lacey, J. H., Crisp, A. H., Kalucy, R. S., Hartmann, M. K., & Chen, C. N. Weight gain and the sleeping electroencephalogram: Study of 10 patients with anorexia nervosa. *British Medical Journal*, 1975, *4*, 556–558.

Lacey, J. H., Stanley, P., Hartmann, M., Koval, J., & Crisp, A. H. The immediate effect of intravenous specific nutrients on EEG sleep. *Electroencephalography and Clinical Neurophysiology*, 1978, *44*, 275–280.

Laird, D. A., & Drexel, H. Experiments with foods and sleep. *Journal of the American Dietetic Association*, 1934, *10*, 89–99.

Lavie, P., Kripke, D. F., Hiatt, J. F., & Harrison, J. Brief report: Gastric rhythms during sleep. *Behavioral Biology*, 1978, *23*, 526–530.

Lawrence, B. E. *A questionnaire and electroencephalographic study of normal napping in a college occupied population*. Unpublished master's thesis, University of Oklahoma, 1971.

Lewis, S. A., Oswald, I., Dunleavy, D. L. F. Chronic fenfluramine administration: Some cerebral effects. *British Medical Journal*, 1971, *3*, 67–70.

Lust, F. Ueber die Beeinflusung der postenzephalitischen Schlafstoerung durch temperatursteigende Mittel. *Deutsche Medizinische Wochenschrift*, 1921, *47*, 1545–1547.

Lutz, E. G. Restless legs, anxiety and caffeinism. *Journal of Clinical Psychiatry*, 1978, *39*, 693–698.

Macho, J. R., & Sinha, A. K. Glucose metabolism during sleep and wakefulness. *Life Sciences*, 1980, *26*, 291–296.

Marks, M. B. Bruxism in allergic children. *American Journal of Orthodontics*, 1980, *77*, 48–59.

Mendelson, W. B., Slater, S., Gold, P., & Gillin, J. C. Changes in human sleep induced by growth hormone administration. *Sleep Research*, 1980, *9*, 93.

Michaelis, R. Depressive Verstimmung and Schlafsucht. *Archiv fur Psychiatrie and Nervenkrankheiten*, 1964, *206*, 345–355.

Neil, J. F., Himmelhoch, J. M., Mallinger, A. G., Mallinger, J., & Hanin, I. Caffeinism complicating hypersomnic depressive episodes. *Comprehensive Psychiatry*, 1978, *19*, 377–385.

Neil, J. F., Merikangas, J. R., Foster, F. G., Merikangas, K. R., Spiker, D. G., & Kupfer, D. J. Waking and all-night sleep EEG's in anorexia nervosa. *Clinical Electroencephalography*, 1980, *11*, 9–15.

Oswald, I., Berger, R. J., Evans, J. I., & Thacore, V. R. Effects of L-tryptophan on human sleep. *Electroencephalography and Clinical Neurophysiology*, 1964, *17*, 603.

Oswald, I., Jones, H. S., & Mannerheim, J. E. Effects of two slimming drugs on sleep. *British Medical Journal*, 1968, *1*, 796–799.

Pavlinac, D., Berman, J., Kripke, D. F., & Deftos, L. Sleep stages effects on plasma minerals. *Sleep Research*, 1978, *7*, 74.

Pfeiffer, C. C., Better nutrition: The practical approach to sleeping better. *The Health Quarterly (Plus Two)*, 1979, *4*, 20–21, 74–75.

Phillips, F., Chen, C. N., Crisp, A. H., Koval, J., McGuinness, B., Kalucy, R. S., Kalucy, E. C., & Lacey, J. H. Isocaloric diet changes and electroencephalographic sleep. *The Lancet*, 1975, *2*, 723–725.

Randolph, T. G. The scope of food and chemical allergy/addiction. *Continuing Education*, September, 1979, pp. 63–76.

Raskind, M. A., & Eisdorfer, C. When elderly patients can't sleep. *Drug Therapy*, August, 1977, pp. 44–50.

Rodden, A., Sinha, A. K., Dement, W. C., Berchas, J. D., Zarcone, V. P., MacLeury, M. R., & De Grazia, J. A. CO_2 elimination from C tyrosine in human sleep and wakefulness. *Brain Research*, 1973, *59*, 427–431.

Rojas-Ramirez, J. A., Shkurovich, M., Ugartechea, J. C., Drucker-Colin, R. R. Evidence supporting a REM sleep–protein relationship, *Sleep Research*, 1976, *5*, 59.

Roth, B. Narcolepsy and hypersomnia. In R. L. Williams & I. Karacan (Eds.), *Sleep disorders: Diagnosis and treatment*. New York: John Wiley & Sons, 1978.

Sitarim, N., Moore, A. M., & Gillin, J. C. Acetylcholine and sleep III: Effect of oral choline on normal human sleep. *Sleep Research*, 1978, *7*, 86.

Southwell, P. R., Evans, C. R., & Hunt, J. N. Effect of hot milk drink on movements during sleep. *British Medical Journal*, 1972, *2*, 429–431.

Spiegel, R. *Sleep and sleeplessness in advanced age*. New York: Spectrum Publications, 1981.

Sugerman, A. A., Southern, D. L., & Rizvi, S. S. H. *In vitro specific IgE measurement: A technique for the discovery of allergic factors in alcoholics, depressives, and schizophrenics*. Paper presented at the Third International Food Allergy Symposium, Boston, October, 1980.

Sullivan, C. E., Henderson-Smart, D. J., & Read, D. J. C. (Eds.). The control of breathing during sleep. *Sleep*, 1980, *3*.

Treichler, F. R., & Hall, J. F. The relationship between deprivation, weight loss and several measures of activity. *Journal of Comparative Physiology and Psychology*, 1962, *55*, 348–349.

Wada, T. Experimental study of hunger in its relation to activity. *Archives of Psychology*, 1922, *8*, 1–65.

Webb, W. B. *Sleep—the gentle tyrant*. Englewood Cliffs, N.J.: Prentice-Hall, 1975.

Weitzman, E. D. (Ed.). *Narcolepsy*. New York: Spectrum Publications, 1976.

Wyatt, R. J., Engleman, K., Kupfer, D. J., Fram, D. H., Sjoerdsma, A., Snyder, F. The effects of L-tryptophan (a natural sedative) on human sleep. *The Lancet*, 1970, *2*, 842–846.

Wyatt, R. J., & Gillin, J. C. Biochemistry and human sleep. In R. L. Williams & I. Karacan (Eds.), *Pharmacology of sleep*. New York: John Wiley & Sons, 1976.

Index